Portraits of Violence

Corporealities: Discourses of Disability

Series editors: David T. Mitchell and Sharon L. Snyder

Recent Titles

Portraits of Violence: War and the Aesthetics of Disfigurement
by Suzannah Biernoff

Bodies of Modernism: Physical Disability in Transatlantic Modernist Literature
by Maren Tova Linett

War on Autism: On the Cultural Logic of Normative Violence
by Anne McGuire

The Biopolitics of Disability: Neoliberalism, Ablenationalism, and Peripheral Embodiment
by David T. Mitchell with Sharon L. Snyder

Foucault and the Government of Disability, Enlarged and Revised Edition
by Shelley Tremain, editor

The Measure of Manliness: Disability and Masculinity in the Mid-Victorian Novel
by Karen Bourrier

American Lobotomy: A Rhetorical History
by Jenell Johnson

Shakin' All Over: Popular Music and Disability
by George McKay

The Metanarrative of Blindness: A Re-reading of Twentieth-Century Anglophone Writing
by David Bolt

Disabled Veterans in History
by David A. Gerber, editor

Mad at School: Rhetorics of Mental Disability and Academic Life
by Margaret Price

Disability Aesthetics
by Tobin Siebers

Stumbling Blocks Before the Blind: Medieval Constructions of a Disability
by Edward Wheatley

Signifying Bodies: Disability in Contemporary Life Writing
by G. Thomas Couser

Concerto for the Left Hand: Disability and the Defamiliar Body
by Michael Davidson

The Songs of Blind Folk: African American Musicians and the Cultures of Blindness
by Terry Rowden

Disability Theory
by Tobin Siebers

Fictions of Affliction: Physical Disability in Victorian Culture
by Martha Stoddard Holmes

Disability in Twentieth-Century German Culture
by Carol Poore

Moving Beyond Prozac, DSM, *and the New Psychiatry: The Birth of Postpsychiatry*
by Bradley Lewis

A complete list of titles in the series can be found at www.press.umich.edu

Portraits of Violence

War and the Aesthetics of Disfigurement

SUZANNAH BIERNOFF

University of Michigan Press
Ann Arbor

Published in the United States of America by the
University of Michigan Press
Printed and bound by CPI Group (UK) Ltd, Croydon, CR0 4YY

2020 2019 2018 2017 4 3 2 1

A CIP catalog record for this book is available from the British Library.

Library of Congress Cataloging-in-Publication data has been applied for.

ISBN: 978-0-472-13029-0 (hardback)
ISBN: 978-0-472-12269-1 (e-book)

Cover photograph: A row of eight facial masks in the American Red Cross Studio for Portrait Masks in Paris, ca. 1918, created for soldiers injured in the First World War. These are partial masks that include prosthetic chins, noses, cheeks, and brows. Some masks feature eyeglasses and moustaches. (Courtesy Archives of American Art, Smithsonian Institution, Anna Coleman Ladd papers.)

Contents

ACKNOWLEDGMENTS vii

Introduction 1

1. The Elusive Portrait 25
2. Aversion: A History 55
3. Repairing War's Ravages 81
4. Flesh Poems 114
5. The Afterlife of Henry Lumley 138

Conclusion 164

NOTES 171

WORKS CITED 197

INDEX 207

Acknowledgments

Many friends and colleagues have played a part in the evolution of this book, providing inspiration, helpful criticism and guidance along the way. Thanks especially to: Jane Tynan, Emma Chambers, Lisa Tickner, Claudia Stein, Roger Cooter, Joanna Bourke, Sander Gilman, Gabriel Koureas, Andrei Pop, Mechtild Widrich, Ana Carden-Coyne and Jane Frances, as well as to LeAnn Fields and the anonymous readers at the University of Michigan Press whose insightful comments on early drafts were invaluable.

The book has its origins in research undertaken during a Wellcome Trust Research Leave Award and several chapters expand on journal articles written during this time. An early version of chapter 4, "Flesh Poems," was published in *Visual Culture in Britain* in 2010; chapter 5 continues a story that began with an article on medical archives and digital culture published in *Photographies* in 2012. Chapter 2 returns to the theme of aversion introduced in "The Rhetoric of Disfigurement in First World War Britain" published in 2011 in *Social History of Medicine.* The book was completed while I was on research leave at Birkbeck, University of London, and for that precious period of undisturbed writing I thank my colleagues in the Department of History of Art.

It would have been impossible to include so many images without the generous support of the Leverhulme Trust through a British Academy Small Grant. Nina Berman, Stuart Griffiths, Timothy Greenfield-Sanders, and Simon Norfolk kindly provided copies of their photographs and permission to reproduce them. I am also very grateful to Andrew Bamji, curator of the Gillies Archives until his retirement in 2011; Paddy Hartley, artistic director of *Project Façade*; Catherine Draycott at Wellcome Images; Simon Chaplin at the Wellcome Library; and Sam Alberti at the Hunterian Museum for responding so generously to my requests for images and information. Alt.text captions for the ebook were produced by Stephanie Rosen and the accessibility team at the University of Michigan Library, making the illustrations accessible to blind and visually impaired readers.

Most of all, I owe a debt of gratitude to John Swettenham, whose ability to make me think more clearly and laugh more often I will always be thankful for.

Introduction

In 2006 the New York–based photographer Nina Berman was approached by *People* magazine to take photographs for a story about a U.S. Marine sergeant, Tyler Ziegel, who had been trapped in his burning truck after a suicide bomber attack on the Iraq-Syria border in December 2004. Ty had been in Brooke Army Medical Centre in San Antonio, Texas, for eighteen months by the time Berman met him, and undergone nineteen operations. His shattered skull and face had needed to be reconstructed; he'd lost an eye, one arm, and three fingers from his other hand. Ty's high school sweetheart and fiancée, Renee Kline, moved to Texas to be with him during his treatment and recovery. For the assignment, Berman met the couple and Ty's mother at Brooke Army and spent several days with them at home in Metamora, Illinois, a few months later. She returned for the wedding in October 2006, and took the photograph reproduced here (figure 1) in a commercial portrait studio on the way to the wedding ceremony at Metamora High School.

In the end, *People* magazine didn't use the photograph, and Berman entered it in the World Press Photo Contest. When *Marine Wedding* won the prize for portraiture, the online response was phenomenal. The photo was viewed by hundreds of thousands of people and became the subject of countless blog posts and comment threads. For many Americans, it is an iconic image of the war in Iraq. Reviewing an exhibition of Berman's photographs at the Jen Bekman Gallery in New York in August 2007, the *New York Times* art critic Holland Cotter remarked that

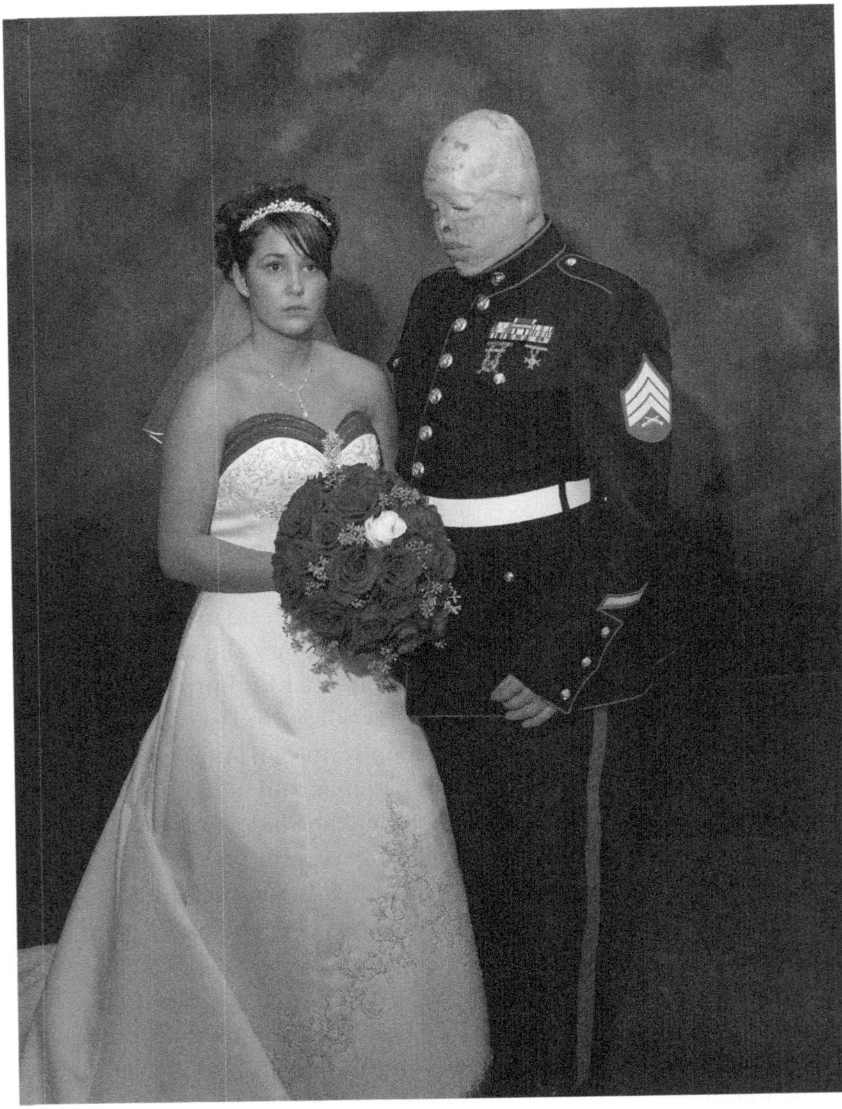

Fig. 1. Nina Berman, *Marine Wedding*, 2006. (© Photo by Nina Berman / NOOR.)

"'Marine Wedding' speaks, as powerfully as a picture can, for itself."[1] But the stream of commentary in the blogosphere suggests otherwise. As Lindsay Beyerstein observed in *Salon*, "Everyone sees something different."[2] *Marine Wedding* was a catalyst. The image, says Berman, "got linked to by everyone from pro-war sites to antiwar sites to sites dedicated to love and Valentine's Day."[3] A copy of the photograph even appeared in the International Triennale of Contemporary Art in 2008, held at the National Gallery in Prague, with the message "Be a hero—marry a hero" obscuring Klein's face.[4] The range of reactions to this one image confirmed what Susan Sontag argued in *Regarding the Pain of Others*: "No 'we' should be taken for granted when the subject is looking at another person's pain."[5]

Sontag's injunction follows her opening discussion of *Three Guineas*, the epistolary essays on war and feminism that Virginia Woolf wrote as a companion piece to her novel *The Years*. Published in 1938, *Three Guineas* begins with an unanswered letter from a peace society: "How in your opinion are we to prevent war?" asks Woolf's unnamed correspondent. In her belated response, Woolf recalls a series of photographs of Spanish civilian casualties taken during the winter of 1936–37:

> This morning's collection contains the photograph of what might be a man's body, or a woman's; it is so mutilated that it might, on the other hand, be the body of a pig. But those certainly are dead children, and that undoubtedly is the section of a house. A bomb has torn open the side; there is still a bird-cage hanging in what was presumably the sitting room.[6]

Photographs like these "are not an argument," Woolf reasons: they are a "crude statement of fact addressed to the eye." Irrespective of class, education, profession, or gender we see "the same picture . . . the same dead bodies, the same ruined houses."[7] We surely share the same horror, she suggests, the same conviction that war must be stopped. For Sontag, though, the imagined photographs are less dependable, their reception and uses less predictable. History tells us that the horrors of war can be used to incite and justify war. Empathy is no more likely a response to such images than rage, or a violent desire for revenge. Pictures—above all those of war and suffering—cannot be depended upon to speak for themselves.

It would be possible to use *Marine Wedding* to ask all kinds of questions: about the medical, military, social, or psychological response to serious combat injuries. These are important issues, but it is equally crucial to interrogate and understand the *representation* of war and injury, because the military body (like the bodies in Woolf's photographs) is more than flesh and blood: it is a symbolic site invested with political as well as personal meaning. Valor, heroism, patriotism, courage: these concepts assume visible form, and do their cultural work, when they are personified and embodied. Mutilated or disabled, the veteran's body can connote the hollowness or corruption of these ideals: a theme most famously exploited in Weimar Germany by the artists aligned with the New Objectivity movement. Such symbolic anatomies have long interested sociologists and anthropologists, who have recognized that the body is a primary system or microcosm of meaning, whether social, political, or cosmological. The sociologist Bryan Turner, for example, suggests that "the dominant concerns and anxieties of society tend to be translated into disturbed images of the body."[8] The mutilated face of war arguably has a special place in this symbolic economy, signifying—perhaps more than any other kind of image—the brutalizing, dehumanizing potential of modern combat.

My own interest in the body and its representations has several origins. The most distant from the subject matter of this book is a doctoral thesis on vision and embodiment in the Middle Ages: a period during which the visual apprehension of (and bodily identification with) abject suffering was promoted as a central tenet of devotional life.[9] Medieval Christians were taught how to look at the mutilated body of Christ: which physical signs of his pain and degradation to dwell on; how to identify with his suffering, what to feel. Familiarity with Christian iconography is by no means irrelevant to the study of twentieth- and twenty-first-century representations of war: together with the classical and Romantic traditions, the conventions of religious art have largely determined the way that death and sacrifice have been imagined and remembered in Western culture. But there is a more profound lesson to be learned from medieval discussions of image devotion. It is that sight itself—as a set of ideas, theories, and experiences—is historical. Scholars of visual culture are sometimes accused of treating images as free-floating signs, abstracted from the material constraints and social contexts of image making and reception.[10] Arguably, though, a genuine interest in the visual (as discourse and practice) should make one more, not less, aware of the material and historical facets of a particular visual object. In this book, my primary concern has been to illuminate the situations in which the injured face was seen, portrayed, and "repaired," not to suggest that the horror of disfigurement is inevitable or historically constant.

A concern with the specific visual encounter has meant that I have privileged the richness of the case study over the appeal of the synoptic overview. With the exception of chapter 2—which deals with the rhetoric of disfigurement—each chapter revolves around a particular image or series of images: *Marine Wedding* is discussed alongside Stuart Griffiths's portraits of British veterans; Henry Tonks's drawings of World War I facial casualties are compared to the medical photographs of the same men in the Gillies Archives; the production of portrait masks for the severely disfigured is approached through the lens of documentary film and photography; and in the final chapter the haunting image of one of Tonks's patients at the Queen's Hospital reappears in the first-person shooter game *BioShock*, provoking an exchange on a players' discussion forum about the ethics of such acts of historical appropriation. This is, then, a study of visual culture rather than a study of art: not just because it includes nonart visual objects (from medical photographs and newspaper clippings to facial casts), but because visual responses to the wounded, disfigured, or disabled body are considered alongside the visual record.

The close analysis of cultural texts or objects is common in literary studies and art history, where issues of context and interpretation are often given more weight than questions of historical continuity or change. It is here that my approach departs from some of the writing that has most inspired and informed it. I am thinking in particular of Joanna Bourke's groundbreaking study of masculinity and the male body in World War I Britain, *Dismembering the Male.* The book's publication in 1996 marked a definitive corporeal turn in World War I studies and has paved the way for subsequent developments in the historiography of the Great War.[11] In the following pages I will plot a genealogy of the wounded body through this family tree, with particular attention to the book that most closely resembles my own in its concern with the *aesthetics* of the damaged and reconstructed body: Ana Carden-Coyne's *Reconstructing the Body: Classicism, Modernism and the First World War* (2009). Other historians have written about the impact of the Great War on literature and the visual arts, but Carden-Coyne follows Bourke in using the wider thematic lens of the body to investigate the extraordinary range of creative responses to the war in Anglophone cultures, from reconstructive surgery and innovations in prosthetics to war memorials, classical revival dance, harmonic gymnastics, bodybuilding, cosmetics and women's fashion. Across these varied cultural arenas, she argues, classicism offered an "aesthetics of healing" as an antidote to the brutal realities of industrialized warfare.[12] In its organization, the book echoes Bourke's thematic chronology of dismembering/remembering. We follow the sudden and shocking unmaking, and more protracted remaking, of the modern body: the body mutilated, dismembered, and obliterated by war; and the body remembered, reconstructed, and reimagined. The most striking difference is the presence of female bodies in the final chapters of *Reconstructing the Body*: slender and athletic or suggestively draped, Carden-Coyne's modern Dianas and Venuses embody the hopes and ideals, and erotic undercurrents, of the interwar years.

The recycling of classical motifs, Carden-Coyne suggests, is not a matter of mere form or rhetoric, but a symptom of much deeper "historical continuities [that] are molded into and performed through the body."[13] The rhetoric of civic virtue, civilization, cultural renewal, and physical perfectibility wasn't new, of course—nor were fears about physical and cultural degeneration—but these ideals and anxieties took on a particular significance for a generation who defined themselves in relation to the experience of mass death and disablement. Turning to the scene of the trauma, Carden-Coyne fleshes out the abject body, interlacing the poetic language of testimonial literature with the cool precision of medical and military history: "Alongside dysentery, pneumonia, and cerebro-spinal disease," for instance, "was the problem of wounds heavily infected with pathogenic organisms, gas gangrene, gas cellulites, and a wide range of foreign bodies such as farmland bacteria, animal excrement, and Mesopotamian dust." Advances in military tactics and weaponry resulted in entirely new kinds of injuries and unforeseen carnage as the "high-speed, rotary motion of [the] dome-tipped bullets reduced the soft tissues and blood vessels to 'a devitalized pulp.'"[14]

Horror can take many forms. By juxtaposing different registers—poetic and scientific, literary and cinematic—Carden-Coyne draws attention to the mediating effects of language and visual culture. She is also alert to the peculiar pull of horror: its powers of fascination (for the spectator anyway) and its uncomfortable proximity to pleasure and desire. The wounded body was a "theatrical site,"[15] the object of civilian curiosity and entertainment, a signifier of authenticity, and a site of memory and mourning. Unusually, the visual forms privileged in this analysis of the war-ravaged body are film, medical images, and literature.[16] Such eclecticism is commonplace in cultural studies and cultural history, but less familiar in disciplines defined by single media (film studies, art history, literature), which typically stress the specificity of their objects (textual, visual, or material) and assume that visual and verbal images are different kinds of things. For Carden-Coyne, war poetry and medical photography are just two examples of the "visual languages of physical suffering that permeated the 'cultural memory' of the war."[17] Methodologically this entails a shift of perspective, away from the particularities of individual sources and toward what has become known as the "cultural imaginary." As with the concept of "cultural transfer," this means pursuing similarities and cultural continuities across different media and in varied social and geographical contexts. Given these ambitions, Carden-Coyne is relatively unconcerned about the possibility of latent meanings or multiple audiences, or the slippery nature of authorial intention—issues that are given more space in Gabriel Koureas's *Memory, Masculinity and National Identity in British Visual Culture, 1914–1930* (2007). Nor does *Reconstructing the Body* excavate the contexts of production and dissemination, the cultural "throw" or impact of individual sources: issues that are addressed more explicitly in this book.[18]

There are passing clues to other narratives in *Reconstructing the Body*; anecdotes and images that can be read against the grain of the central argument. For example, while it is true that World War I was a "highly visual war," the visual experience of death and injury was both partial and policed. As early as November 1914 *The War Illustrated* admitted that "from the pictorial point of view modern warfare lacks much which the battlefields of the past provided. Soldiers today are fighting enemies on the continent whom they never see. . . . For this reason the great mass of photographs which reach us do not show actual hostilities."[19] Visual disorientation—an *inability* to see because traumatized, injured, or groping in the dark—was a defining condition of the western front, as Santanu Das reveals in his moving account of the poetics of touch in World War I literature. Touch, Das suggests, was "the more apt register" when recording the mud, slime, and darkness of the trenches, the immediacy of death and putrefaction and pain.[20] Press censorship (and self-censorship), the selective representation of casualties, the conditions of trench warfare, literary and artistic meditations on the unrepresentability of modern war: these things are evidence of a highly ambivalent and mediated visuality. Facial injury is a case in point. Particularly dreaded by soldiers and their loved ones, facial mutilation was the subject of vivid journalistic writing and extensive medical documentation. But it was almost never illustrated in the wartime press; mirrors were banned from facial wards, and disfigured veterans were socially stigmatized. Carden-Coyne makes the point that suffering and disability were not uniformly represented, but the thrust of her argument privileges the "spectacular" forms of sacrifice and bodily reconstruction rather than the evidence for aversion and censorship.

Was classicism therapeutic? Can we weigh the scales of history and decide whether the cult of health and beauty was liberating or normalizing, pleasurable or oppressive? The problem here—and for cultural historians generally—is that it is extremely difficult to answer psychological questions about people who are dead. As soon as we start asking how people "felt"—what their beliefs and experiences and "imaginaries" were—we have to grapple with what we mean by those things. Do we mean how they wrote about what they felt? Is the history of the body necessarily a history of discourse, representations, signs? "Real bodies," writes Carden-Coyne, "are living interpretations of the visual world of bodily signs,"[21] but I am not convinced that the fissure between lived experience and representation can be so easily mended, not when signs are all that remain of the past.

Reconstructing the Body and the other studies I have touched on here are fine examples of corporeal history. In each case the body is taken as a primary site of "imagination" and "experience" (Bourke's twin foci) in order to challenge assumptions about the impact of the war on collective and individual identities; each can be read, at the same time, as an attempt to reconceptualize embodiment in light of psychoanalytic and poststructuralist theories. When Bourke was writing *Dismembering the Male*, she noted that research on the Great War was dominated by conventional military history, economic history, and literary studies.[22] Social and cultural historians have succeeded in redressing the balance, and it is no longer the case that our knowledge of men's bodies (or women's) in the nineteenth and early twentieth centuries "remains sketchy."[23]

For those interested in the cultural history of World War I, *Portraits of Violence* can be read as a further contribution to this collective project. It, too, deals with the corporeal territories of war as imagined and experienced, although "experience" in this case refers primarily to the public and professional response to disfiguring injury rather than the experience of those who were wounded. There are several other ways in which this book differs from the studies mentioned above, one of the most significant being my decision to include contemporary representations of war, from *Marine Wedding* to the dystopian carnage of *BioShock*. These images do more than make the rhetorical point that our interest in the past has everything to do with the present, although it is a point worth making. Berman's portraits, and those of British veterans by Stuart Griffiths, are included here because they point to the persistence of certain images and themes, such as the virtues of bravery and stoicism and the redemptive power of love (implicitly heterosexual and preferably domestic). It is crucial that we recognize the resilience of such tropes, and their social and political utility. On the other hand, there are significant variations in how, and in what circumstances, the human cost of war has been depicted, and differences too in the medical and social response to disfiguring or disabling injury, as well as people's belief in (or skepticism about) medical progress. Horror—of disfigurement, of war—is a cultural formation. The juxtaposition of historical and contemporary sources is not meant to imply that the face of war is a universal trope; rather, it is a way of allowing questions to surface that might otherwise go unexplored. How and why do these images speak to contemporary concerns? To what extent have attitudes toward disability and disfigurement changed over the last century?

It has become common to speak of the "medical" and "social" models of disability as though they are clear alternatives: either disability is a treatable condition; or it is a socially determined and negotiated idea. Definitions of the social model tend to stress environmental, organizational, and attitudinal barriers to inclusion rather than placing the onus on the individual or the family to seek a medical solution (or on the medical profession to come up with a cure).[24] Advocates of the social model insist that the "problem" is not the disability; "the problem is the way that normalcy is constructed to create the 'problem' of the disabled person."[25] A content analysis of 8,650 hours of television conducted by researchers at Cardiff University in 2006–7 found that disfigurement was often portrayed as "an individual 'problem' that can be solved with biomedical, technological or practical solutions."[26] One of the recurring themes in audience focus groups was the belief that disfigurement was a "last taboo," despite (or perhaps because of) the "current obsession with appearance on television"[27]—the point being that the medical model is inextricably entangled with social attitudes and cultural representations. The surgical and prosthetic "repair" of mutilated faces and shattered limbs was, as we shall see, never a purely medical concern.

Another way in which this book departs from the substantial literature on the Great War is in its sustained attention to the face and portraiture. Bourke focuses on limb loss on the grounds that "the decisive impact of the Great War on men's bodies can be seen most clearly by looking at the war-maimed."[28] Koureas addresses the aesthetics of the male body more directly and touches on the production of portrait masks, but for the main part "masculinity" is located in the discourses of class conflict and commemoration.[29] Carden-Coyne evokes the appalling visibility of the mutilated face and its impact on the "cultural memory" of World War I.[30] She is absolutely right to draw attention to the generalized "'culture shock' of modern warfare" and the theatrical visualization (and sometimes sexualization) of the wounded body, but I would suggest that the injured body was not an undifferentiated symbolic site. As I argue in chapter 2, the relative absence of facial injury from the public visual culture of the war suggests a culture of aversion, not one of display.

*

The social and cultural significance of the face is often overlooked in accounts of the body, gender, and sexuality, and if faces do appear—in portraits or caricatures, for example—they are rarely commented upon. The marginalization of the face in histories of the body is all the more puzzling when one reflects on the central importance of identity and subjectivity in this literature, and the fact that in our everyday lives we habitually rely on the face—often in the absence of any other information—as a signifier of both. The cover image of Mariam Fraser and Monica Greco's *The Body: A Reader* (2005) conveys this peculiar absence well. A black-and-white self-portrait by the Finnish American photographer Arno Rafael Minkkinen, the figure (what little we see of it) comprises two arms, seen from the front, and the broad arc of a back we presume to be the artist's. In a conventional portrait the subject's elbows might be propped on a tabletop, chin in hands: a pose suggestive of intimacy or reverie. Here, the figure's elbows stand directly on the bare floor, and his sinuous hands and forearms cover a dark void where the head should be.

In their introduction, Fraser and Greco quote Bryan Turner's admission (in 1984 when the first edition of *The Body and Society* was published) that he was "increasingly less sure of what the body is." He elaborates with a list of paradoxical truths:

> The body is a material organism, but also a metaphor; it is the trunk apart from the head and limbs, but also the person (as in "anybody" and "somebody"). The body may also be an aggregate of bodies, often with legal personality as in "corporation" or in "the mystical body of Christ." Such aggregate bodies may be regarded as legal fictions or as social facts which exist independently of the "real" bodies which happen to constitute them.[31]

As *The Body: A Reader* makes abundantly clear, the potential topics for students of this new sub- or transdiscipline are even more expansive than the answers to the question, what is a body? Organ transplants, imperial advertising, reproductive technologies, aging and embodiment, the concept of "genetic risk," images of disability, the body as consumer object, craniometry, cross-dressing, the body in pain, AIDS portraits, lesbian bodies, the biology of sexual difference, the Visible Human Project, Roman and early Christian bodies, the histories of the monstrous and grotesque: the possibilities are probably limitless. Greco and Fraser are sociologists, but many of the texts they include in their anthology have been foundational in other disciplines as well: from Mary Douglas's *Natural Symbols* (1970) and Michel Foucault's *Discipline and Punish* (1979) to Judith Butler's *Bodies That Matter* (1993) and Elaine Scarry's *The Body in Pain* (1985). Within this porous interdisciplinary field, the face has tended to be approached in one of three ways: through the history of the photographic portrait; in relation to aesthetic and reconstructive surgery; and more recently, as a vehicle for exploring ideas of ugliness, monstrosity and the grotesque. Although not thematized as such by Fraser and Greco, there are examples of all three approaches in their reader.

The first category is represented by excerpts from Allan Sekula's "The Body and the Archive," a seminal work of Foucauldian historiography. Published in the journal *October* in 1986, the essay charts the emergence and instrumental potential of the photographic portrait: a "system of representation," Sekula explains, that was effective precisely because it was "capable of functioning both *honorifically* and *repressively*":

> On the one hand, the photographic portrait extends, accelerates, popularizes, and degrades a traditional function. This function, which can be said to have taken its early modern form in the seventeenth century, is that of providing for the ceremonial presentation of the bourgeois *self*. . . . At the same time, photographic portraiture began to perform a role no painted portrait could have performed in the same thorough and rigorous fashion. This role derived, not from any honorific portrait tradition, but from the imperatives of medical and anatomical illustration. Thus photography came to establish and delimit the terrain of the *other*.[32]

Every portrait—the cherished memento of a loved one no less than a police mug shot—placed its subject "within a social and moral hierarchy."[33] Photography thus became an indispensable and extremely subtle instrument of social surveillance (and more importantly *self*-surveillance): a technological extension of the anonymous and continuous gaze of the panopticon.[34] For Foucault, Jeremy Bentham's "perfect" prison was a chilling metaphor for the modern disciplinary society in which the condition of total visibility had replaced physical restraint, functioning as a "trap" and a "guarantee of order."[35] Building on Foucault's account, Sekula argues that photography came to define both the "*generalized look*" (the typology) and the "*contingent instance* of deviance and social pathology."[36] The result was a new vision of society as a vast "shadow archive" in which the "traces of the visible bodies of heroes, leaders, moral exemplars, celebrities" lined up with "those of the poor, the diseased, the insane, the criminal, the nonwhite, the female, and all other embodiments of the unworthy."[37]

This fantasy of an all-encompassing and empirically verifiable social taxonomy was not entirely new. Photography's instrumental appeal was based, in part, on the prior claims of physiognomy and phrenology, "sciences" that attempted to use facial features (in the case of physiognomy) or cranial topography (in phrenology) as a measurable index of character and intelligence. These ideas had been around for a very long time,[38] but the revival of physiognomy toward the end of the eighteenth century has been linked to the demographic changes precipitated by the Industrial Revolution. As cities became more populous and people more mobile, contact with strangers—and with "difference" in all its guises—became an everyday experience; especially with the advent of illustrated papers and other mass media. The idea that the most visible, most public part of human anatomy, the face, could be systematically classified and interpreted helped to ameliorate the experience of rapid social change. As Sekula remarks: "Here was a method for quickly assessing the character of strangers in the dangerous and congested spaces of the nineteenth-century city. Here was a gauge of the intentions and capabilities of the other."[39] Although the scientific credibility of physiognomy had waned by the end of the nineteenth century, its influence persists even today in visual representations of class, gender, and race (not least in the context of war, where the face of the enemy often conforms to physiognomic stereotypes). The conviction that "all society's ills are *visible*"—to quote Richard Sennett—is no less prevalent today than it was a century ago.[40]

Both portraiture and physiognomy rely on the premise that the face is a reliable index of gender, age, social and familial identity, ethnicity, emotion, and much more besides. However, beneath the face we are meat, a fact that artists like Henry Tonks and Francis Bacon reveal only too well. Physiognomy's "perceptual agenda" breaks down in the presence of the mutilated or surgically altered face.[41] The surgeon Harold Delf Gillies (1882–1960) describes the sight, following the Somme, of "men burned and maimed to the condition of animals."[42] Faces register emotion and identity, but they are also conventional markers of the boundary between the human and the nonhuman, and between "civilization and barbarism."[43] From Pliny's monstrous races to Christopher Nolan's *The Dark Knight,* we find facial disfigurement signifying a loss or deficit of human nature, a loss that as a narrative trope often prefigures a character's death.[44]

In Fraser and Greco's anthology we are given a glimpse of the vertiginous *in*humanity of the face in the "carnal art" of the French performance and multimedia artist Orlan. Best known for nine "surgery-performances" between 1990 and 1993, Orlan has described her body as "a place of public debate"[45] and warned her audience during the operations (broadcast around the world live via video link), "You are about to see videos which will make you suffer."[46] The convention of the before and after photograph has been exploited by plastic surgeons since the 1840s, but Orlan is interested in surgery itself as a theatrical site and rite of passage.[47] Her desire to "show that which is usually kept secret" extended to the documentation of her bruised and swollen postoperative face, first thing in the morning, every morning, for forty-one days, while the sale of "relics" (vials of blood and fluids) for $100 pushed the rhetoric of artist as commodity to its ironic conclusion.[48] As an art history student in the early 1990s, I watched Orlan's surgical "reincarnation" with a mixture of skepticism and fascination. Two details remain vivid. One is an image from her seventh operation, *Omnipresence* (1993), in which a flap of skin hangs open beneath her left ear as she turns to look over her right shoulder, chin slightly raised, features composed into a perfect profile. There is the visceral jolt of seeing raw flesh beneath the skin of the face, but what really shocks is the sudden realization that the face is a seperable thing: a piece of skin that can be simply peeled away. Portraiture is usually conceived as the *representation* of the face: Orlan shows us the face *as* portrait.

My other enduring memory is of the artist's voice. *Omnipresence* was transmitted live to audiences in New York, Paris, Toronto, Banff, and eleven other cities around the world. While the surgeon Marjorie Cramer inserted implants into her chin and temples, Orlan read aloud from Lemoine-Luccioni's *La Robe* and answered questions via fax from the audience. As Parveen Adams later wrote, it was as though her body was "surgically severed from speech."[49] Orlan has described the physical body as "obsolete" and "no more than a bag."[50] Her performances stage the disturbance, if not demise, of the "natural" body in an era of rapid and profound biotechnological change. But what remains, for Orlan, as an unbroken signifier of agency and subjectivity, is the voice. Language as skin, although not as Roland Barthes imagined it, trembling with desire:[51] Orlan's is not a voice that caresses or cuts; it is the voice as protective membrane, an organ that contains and communicates the "self." While it would be wrong to overemphasize the similarities between these postmodern surgery-performances and the evolving "art" of reconstructive surgery, there is something about the interaction of voice and face that deserves closer attention. "If you closed your eyes," says Berman of Ziegel, "you would feel he was a completely healthy person."[52] When the subjective voice (spoken or written) is absent—as it typically is in medical representations—it is difficult to see past the visual record of injury, disfigurement, or disease. Conversely, personal narratives are often used (by Berman among others) to humanize images of trauma, and to counteract or compensate for the objectifying and "othering" effects of photography.

Sander Gilman's *Making the Body Beautiful: A Cultural History of Aesthetic Surgery* is not one of the texts in Fraser and Greco's anthology, although it would have made a provocative historical counterpoint to Orlan's "carnal art." It is, however, one of the few books to focus on the cultural history of the face, and an indispensable reference work for anyone interested in the history of plastic surgery. With particular attention to the nose, Gilman considers the history and meaning of aesthetic surgery through an array of popular and literary sources as well as medical texts and images. From its beginnings in the 1890s, modern aesthetic surgery was understood as a way of mitigating difference: first racial difference (the "African," "Oriental," or "Jewish" nose) and then an ever-expanding catalog of bodily differences. Surgery held the promise of bodily transformation, and with it passage from one social category to another: from old to youthful; undesirable to desirable; pathological to normal; and ultimately from unhappy to happy. "What remains constant," Gilman explains, "is the idea that the external body (with whatever qualities are ascribed to it) reflects the values of the soul."[53] The history of plastic surgery is inseparable from the parallel history of physiognomy and its insidious "perceptual agenda," but it also gives form to the idea that we are made (and maintained) rather than born; that beauty is an aspiration and an imperative, something you work at and invest in, rather than simply a gift of nature.

The rhetoric of aesthetic enhancement and personal realization is complicated by the case of war surgery, to which Gilman devotes a chapter. For those whose faces were mutilated on the battlefields of the Great War, "passing" as normal was not an option: the most one could hope for was to be restored to "somewhat human" form.[54] The "missing face," Gilman suggests, "could only be understood as a loss of humanity."[55] It is here—at the supposed corporeal limits of the human—that descriptions of facial injury and disfigurement exploit the language of the monstrous. The monstrous, and its sibling the grotesque, are ideas with long histories and manifold uses, and it is helpful to establish some preliminary definitions before we encounter these terms in their twentieth-century incarnations. "Monstrous births" (human and animal) and "monstrous races" first appear as objects of scientific and religious speculation in classical literature.[56] For medieval commentators they were demonstrations (from the Latin *monstrum*, meaning portent) of the genetic wages of sin: a belief that extended from morphological anomalies ("monstrous births") to the devastating effects of diseases like leprosy.[57] Deformities of all kinds—whether congenital or acquired—were taken as signs of moral and intellectual degeneracy. "Evil men lose their identity," explained Roger Bacon in his thirteenth-century treatise on moral philosophy, "because the identity of a thing consists in retaining its order and preserving its nature." Because sin "is contrary to the order of nature . . . you cannot regard as a human being the man whom you see transformed by vices."[58]

In the early modern period, monsters populated scholarly discussions of natural philosophy and law; they were displayed at fairs; featured in religious pamphlets; and represented in the woodcuts and ballads that preceded newspapers. In their study of sixteenth- and seventeenth-century monster literature in England and France, Katherine Park and Lorraine Daston trace the evolution of "monsters" from divine prodigies (where they appear alongside natural disasters, celestial apparitions, and portentous rains of blood and stones) to "natural wonders—signs of nature's fertility rather than God's wrath."[59] By the eighteenth century the "monster" had lost its apocalyptic associations, along with its ability to inspire wonder, and had begun to be incorporated into the new medical specialisms of comparative anatomy and embryology. Despite the secularization and medicalization of what Rosemarie Garland-Thomson calls "the extraordinary body," "freaks of nature" continued to be displayed in fairgrounds and museums well into the twentieth century; indeed, documentaries like Channel 4's *Body Shock* strand rely on an undiminished fascination with extremes of human embodiment.[60] Anomalous, extraordinary, or just curiously different: these are bodies onto which our collective "anxieties, questions, and needs" might be projected "at any given moment."[61]

There is an important difference, however, between the early modern "appetite for the marvellous" (which the philosopher David Hume regarded as the hallmark of the "ignorant and barbarous") and its late modern equivalents.[62] In the marketplace and the fairground "monsters" and "freaks" were never presented as objects of pity. The intermingling of fascination with *pity* (as distinct from terror, wonder, or amusement) is a modern development, coinciding with the rise of humanitarianism, the professionalization of charities, and the institutionalization of people with physical disabilities. As the sociologist Robert Bogdan argues in *Freakery: Cultural Spectacles of the Extraordinary Body*, "Pity combined with the medical model became the dominant mode of presenting human differences for money. It is through this lens that we look back on freak shows and find them distasteful."[63] During the Great War, the horror of disfigurement was almost always accompanied by pity for its "victim" or his family, and both horror and pity were part of the stock-in-trade of charitable fund-raising. Yet the old idea of the "monster" as a portent is there as well: a demonstration not of sin or divine displeasure, but of the apocalyptic nature of war.

The terms "grotesque" and "monstrous" are often used interchangeably, but the grotesque has acquired a particular currency in literary and cultural theory of the last thirty years, where it is linked to the politics of transgression.[64] The key text here is Mikhail Bakhtin's *Rabelais and His World*, an account of medieval and Renaissance folk humor and the "carnivalesque."[65] Bakhtin's definition of the grotesque body includes one of the very few descriptions of facial features in Fraser and Greco's anthology:

> Of all the features of the human face, the nose and mouth play the most important part in the grotesque image of the body. . . . The eyes have no part in these comic images; they express an individual, so to speak, self-sufficient human life, which is not essential to the grotesque.[66]

For Bakhtin, the grotesque body and its polar twin, the classical body, function at the level of signification. They are unstable categories through which the dominant term (classical, civilization, beauty) continually defines itself in opposition to an other.[67] Accordingly, "The artistic logic of the grotesque image ignores the closed, smooth, and impenetrable surface of the body and retains only its excrescences (sprouts, buds) and orifices, only that which leads beyond the body's limited space or into the body's depths."[68] While there are intriguing parallels between Bakhtin's description of grotesque bodily imagery and the spectacle of war-damaged bodies, some caution is required. Bakhtin's grotesque bodies were comic, not tragic; and they were visible—part of a thriving folk culture—not institutionalized. The grotesque, as Bakhtin understood it, is not a transhistorical category. There are, he claims, "no signs of duality" in the modern body: which is to say, the "excrescences" and "depths" of the modern body are no longer public and visible but private and psychological.[69] They are also medical, of course: birth, death, the signs of aging, and the regulation of our bodies' daily functions are understood within a medical paradigm that did not exist before the nineteenth century. When we encounter the "mournful grotesquerie" of the war wounded, it is in the ward of a London hospital.[70] The operating theater and hospital ward are two of the places where the "duality" of the modern body is revealed, and it is here that one finds, perhaps, a survival of the comic grotesque, in the memoirs and diaries of nurses, doctors, and orderlies.

*

This book explores the idea and image of disfigurement in one of its most troubling modern formations, as a symbol and consequence of industrialized war. Chapter 1 returns to the scene of *Marine Wedding* and Berman's earlier series, *Purple Hearts*, in order to probe the conventions and limits of portraiture as a means of conveying the human cost of war. We speak of giving war or suffering a "human face," but in Berman's work the social and psychological effects of armed conflict are signified by the destruction of the recognizably human form. The relationship between portraiture and trauma is further elaborated through the work of Stuart Griffiths, a British photographer and former paratrooper who has spent a decade documenting the experiences of homeless and disabled ex-service personnel. Both Berman and Griffiths have spoken eloquently about the personal as well as the political nature of their work (Berman in public talks and interviews; Griffiths in the 2009 documentary *Isolation*, directed by Luke Seomore and Joseph Bull). All portraits involve processes of social and aesthetic negotiation. Often unspoken, these subtleties are lost when we speak of a portrait as a "good likeness": a concept that runs aground when the subject of the portrait has suffered psychological damage or life-changing injury, and that disavows the mediated nature of all representations. The questions posed in this first chapter provide a conceptual foundation for the book as a whole. What is a portrait? How does trauma (physical or psychological) alter or transform the genre of portraiture?

Chapter 2 considers the stigma of disfigurement during World War I. In wartime Britain (the geographical focus of this study) the horror of facial mutilation was evoked in journalism, poems, memoirs, and fiction; but it was almost never represented visually outside the professional contexts of clinical medicine and medical history. There are medical representations of facial injury from the Battle of Waterloo (a remarkable series of watercolors by the surgeon and anatomist Sir Charles Bell),[71] and photographs from the American Civil War,[72] but the men wounded in those conflicts were unlikely to live with severely disfiguring injuries. The steel helmet—first used by British troops in 1916—decreased the number of fatal head injuries, but left the face itself exposed to snipers and flying shell fragments. New types of guns and ammunition, produced on an industrial scale, inflicted more damage—and more complex wounds—than those caused by ordinary rifles. At the medical museum attached to Val-de-Grâce Hospital in Paris, visitors could marvel at the foreign objects extracted from the faces of the patients: "shell caps almost intact, five franc pieces bent into all sorts of shapes, lumps of lead inches thick and many horrid, ragged pieces of shell which play havoc with the flesh, bullets, bits of uniform, even long lengths of material."[73] Severely disfigured servicemen were considered unfit for active duty because of the effect of their appearance on morale, and facial injury was consistently described in the wartime press as an unimaginable tragedy.[74] "What kind of vision does your mind conjure up when you hear or see the word 'wounded?'" begins an article in the British tabloid *Daily Sketch*:

> Probably, if you are an average stay-at-home civilian, a limping man in a blue hospital suit or, at worst, an indefinite huddled figure on a stretcher. But there are other wounded that the mind instinctively avoids contemplating. There are men who come from battle still walk-

> ing firmly, still with capable hands, unscarred bodies, but who are the most tragic of all war's victims, whose endurance is to be tried in the hardest days, who are now half strangers among their own people, and reluctant even to tread the long-wished-for paths of home. In medical language they are classed as "Facial and Jaw Cases." Think that phrase over for a minute and realise what it may mean.[75]

Journalists invariably praised the miraculous work of surgeons like Harold Gillies, but the story of medical progress did not easily translate into images. Nor was the mutilated and disfigured body of the war veteran exploited as a site of collective shame or trauma in Anglophone cultures the way it was in Weimar Germany.[76] There was no British or American equivalent to Otto Dix or Max Beckmann. Rather than dwelling on the causes or consequences of war, English art of the 1920s was characterized by "retreat, evasion, and concealment of modernity's impact."[77] In this respect, Bryan Turner's observation that social anxieties tend to be manifest in images of bodily disorder needs some qualification: historically these have often been the very images subject to censure. Disfigurement and disability become politically charged when they connote a loss that cannot be overcome or compensated. If we compare the rhetoric of disfigurement to portrayals of limb loss, an asymmetrical picture emerges in which the "worst loss of all"—the loss of one's face—is perceived as a loss of humanity.

The most detailed narrative account of facial injury and its treatment in wartime Britain is in Ward Muir's *The Happy Hospital*, which was published in 1918. A corporal in the Royal Army Medical Corps, Muir had written several novels before the war as well as occasional pieces for magazines. He also edited *Happy—Though Wounded*, a fund-raising publication with contributions from staff and patients at the Third London General Hospital, drawn from the hospital's *Gazette*. We encounter the facial ward in the final chapter of Muir's otherwise upbeat portrait of hospital life. It is "something of an ordeal," he writes:

> To talk to a lad who, six months ago, was probably a wholesome and pleasing specimen of English youth, and is now a gargoyle, and a broken gargoyle at that,—the only decent features remaining being perhaps one eye, one ear, and a shock of boyish hair. . . . You know very well that he has examined himself in a mirror. That one eye of his has contemplated the mangled mess which is his face—all the more hopeless because "healed." . . . He is aware of just what he looks like:

> therefore you feel intensely that he is aware that you are aware, and that some unguarded glance of yours may cause him hurt. This, then, is the patient at whom you are afraid to gaze unflinchingly: not afraid for yourself, but for *him.*[78]

One of the few exceptions to the tacit censorship of facial injury in wartime Britain is a series of photographs taken by the official home front photographer Horace Nicholls, documenting the making and fitting of a prosthetic mask. As I argue in chapter 3, these are ambiguous images that blur the line between photojournalism, art photography, and official record-keeping. Like most of Nicholls's photographs for Wellington House (the British government's propaganda bureau), the series he captioned "Repairing War's Ravages" seems to have remained unseen by the public. The two young men whose reconstruction he documents are stoical and self-composed, their "repair" (under the watchful eye of the sculptor Francis Derwent Wood) is seemingly flawless; yet it is hard to imagine the photographs featuring in a propaganda campaign. As much as the sculptor's skill they evoke the loss of identity alluded to in written accounts.

Wood was not the only sculptor involved in this work. Kathleen Scott (the widow of Captain Robert Falcon Scott and one of Henry Tonks's former students at the Slade) worked at the Ellerman Hospital for officers in Regent's Park, and wrote in her diary that it made her feel "terribly like God, the creator."[79] Anna Coleman Ladd, an American sculptor, opened her own Studio for Portrait Masks in Paris in late 1917, under the auspices of the American Red Cross and in consultation with Derwent Wood. Ladd's American, French, and British team included three sculptors, two of them women (Jane Poupelet and Louise Brent). When Ladd's husband, a prominent Boston pediatrician, was appointed to head the Children's Bureau of the American Red Cross in Toul, she embraced her own project with vigor: filling the large artist's studio in the Latin Quarter with flowers, posters, and French and American flags, as well as casts of masks in progress.[80] A silent film made for the American Red Cross documents Ladd and her assistants at work. The two *mutilés de guerre* featured in the short film seem entirely at ease with the attention they are receiving. One smiles, chats and smokes a cigarette for the camera as Ladd admires his new chin from different angles. The social intimacy and informality of the scene suggest that in this context at least the stigma of facial injury was not insurmountable.[81]

The most sustained artistic response to facial injury, however, is the series of pastel drawings by Henry Tonks (1862–1937) of soldiers before and after facial reconstructive surgery. Tonks had been a surgeon before his celebrated career as an artist and teacher at the Slade School of Art in London, and these intimate studies—the focus of chapter 4—lie somewhere between medical illustrations and portraits. Never intended for public exhibition, they nonetheless raise questions about the proximity of art and science—and beauty and horror—that transcend their original function. A selection was displayed in 2002 alongside photographs and case histories in the Strang Print Room gallery at University College London. In June 2007, the full series was made available on the website of the Gillies Archives.[82] Renewed interest in the cultural history of medicine has coincided, in the UK, with a number of major exhibitions and art/science projects, and Tonks has emerged as a recurring presence. In the Science Museum's *Future Face* exhibition in 2004, the Tonks pastels were used to make a point about the absence of the disfigured face from traditional portraiture. In *War and Medicine* at Wellcome Collection and *Faces of Battle* at the National Army Museum, artistic and scientific responses to the war-damaged body were deliberately juxtaposed.[83] The crossing of disciplinary boundaries in this book—from art to medical illustration, from the history of surgery to popular culture—has a rather different motivation. When curators put art objects in a room with objects that are not art, it is invariably art's role to illustrate, illuminate, or provoke; to answer a perceived need for visual explanation or contemplation.[84] Derwent Wood's portrait masks, Nicholls's photographs, and Tonks's pastel studies fulfill these requirements well, but they are included here for another reason. These fragile, intimate objects are evidence that being human (in the sense of creating, preserving, or restoring "humanity") is a cultural and aesthetic matter as much as a biological or medical one. In *Sites of Memory, Sites of Mourning* Jay Winter describes the aesthetic response to the collective slaughter of the Great War as a response to "symbolic collapse."[85] The idea of symbolic collapse comes from Julia Kristeva's study of depression and melancholia and becomes, in turn, an organizing concept for Winter's book.[86] As he explains:

> "Symbolic collapse" threatened all those who tried to understand the meaning of loss of life in the Great War. Art and ceremony helped shore up these symbols, through which grief was expressed and bereavement experienced. Following Kristeva, we can see how it was not only individuals, therefore, but also the symbols of meaning which were "resurrected" during and after the war.[87]

Winter focuses on the loss of life and on literary, artistic, and architectural forms of commemoration, mourning, and "redemption,"[88] but there were other memories, other losses for which there was no older language, no ceremonial tradition or "sublimatory solution."[89] When medical archives document the horrors of war, they can be particularly difficult to contemplate because they connect us to events and experiences that can seem, to quote the British painter Paul Nash, "utterly indescribable."[90] The interlinked case studies in this book are responses to a "symbolic collapse" as profound as the loss of life, but much harder to grieve for.

Chapter 5 returns us to the present by investigating the digital resurrection of one of Gillies's patients in the computer game *BioShock*. When *BioShock* was released by 2K Games in August 2007, reviewers praised its dystopian vision of modernity and the moral complexities of the plot. What critics overlooked was the extent to which the disturbingly realistic artwork and musical score relied on found images and sound, including a recording of distressed breathing from a doctor's website, and digitized World War I medical photographs from the Gillies Archives. There has been very little discussion about the ethical implications of such acts of commercial and creative appropriation, despite the increasing availability of historical archives online and the popularity of collections and events that explore the "interstices" between medicine and art.[91] When Tonks's surgical portraits, or the photographs in the Gillies Archives, cross the tenuous line dividing "science" from "art"—or stray beyond their original diagnostic, documentary, or didactic context—they begin to ask questions of *us*. To what extent are our responses to the damaged body universal—or culturally learned and regulated within specific contexts of viewing? How does one, might one, should one, look at images of the body in pain? The final chapter provides a critical framework for these crucial questions and considers the broader significance of historical representation and context in contemporary art and digital culture.

Each of the scenarios examined in this book corroborates Rosemarie Garland-Thomson's argument that "the extraordinary body is fundamental to the narratives by which we make sense of ourselves and our world."[92] In *BioShock*, the surgically and genetically "enhanced" inhabitants of Rapture demonstrate the grotesque consequences of a world where physical perfection has become a moral imperative. For Henry Tonks and Francis Derwent Wood, surgical and prosthetic "repair" were the only hope of salvation for men whose injuries compromised their very identity. In every case discussed here, the body is socially negotiated and culturally mediated: not just through discourses (of sacrifice, repair, and redemption, for example), but perceptually too. In *Staring: How We Look*, Garland-Thomson corrects the objectifying bias of many accounts of disability by attending to the dynamics of intense looking: "how staring works, what it does, and how it makes us who we are."[93] Before we look more closely at the contemporary portraiture of war, it is worth reflecting on the value of these questions for the historical study of stigma.

The gaze has become a familiar term in art history, film theory, and visual studies, denoting a sexualized ("male gaze"), dehumanizing ("medical gaze"), or disciplinary mode of vision. As a concept, the gaze encompasses changing technologies and styles of representation—from microscopy to medical photography, Hollywood cinema to CCTV—as well as ways of looking. What these practices have in common is an assumed asymmetry: the gaze implies an object; and that object (the female body, the disease, the criminal) is denied the possibility of looking back. For Garland-Thomson, staring is more complicated than this. She sets out to unsettle "common understandings that staring is rudeness, voyeurism, or surveillance or that starers are perpetrators and starees victims." What interests her is "staring's generative potential."[94] She explores what it is like to be regarded with curiosity, amazement, or horror, but also how those with "stareable traits" manage these highly charged visual interactions.

Garland-Thomson's privileging of autobiographical sources (including a questionnaire completed by thirty-five people with visible disabilities) allows her to approach staring as a complex interaction rather than a one-way street. As a primary manifestation of the stigmatizing process, staring disrupts the "effortless mutual granting of civil inattention that gets us through our day."[95] It can be an intensely uncomfortable experience for the starer too, because staring brings us face to face with our own "ontological contingency . . . the truth of our body's vulnerability to the randomness of fate."[96] Perfect health and physical attractiveness are, at best, temporary states of being: sooner or later we all experience impairment, disability, or dependence, if only because we get sick or grow old.

In the United States, where Garland-Thomson lives and works, and in Britain and Australia, the countries I am most familiar with, disability has a precarious visibility: "care in the community" can be a euphemism for social isolation; the aged and severely disabled are sequestered in residential facilities; illness is medicalized, death institutionalized; and "normality" is the subject of relentless definition.[97] "When we do see the usually concealed sight of disability writ boldly on others," writes Garland-Thomson, "we stare in fascinated disbelief and uneasy identification. Why, we ask with our eyes, does that person with dwarfism, that amputee, that drooler, look so much like and yet so different from me?"[98] Media and sporting events like the London 2012 Paralympic Games have given us positive images of disability, but to qualify as "Superhuman" you need to be young, athletic, and extraordinarily determined.[99] Endurance, courage, strength, resilience, optimism: these are the character traits that, as communities, we make visible and celebrate. Those who cannot overcome their obstacles—or choose not to—more often provoke pity, embarrassment, or anger.

Staring: How We Look is not intended as a cultural history. Garland-Thomson describes it as an "anatomy" of staring, but at its core is a question of ethics: not how *do* we stare (a question for social scientists and psychologists) or how has staring been understood and regulated in the past (a historian might have a shot at that), but rather how *should* we stare?[100] The mutual discomfort of staring, she suggests, can "beget mutual recognition" and even open our eyes to beauty of another order. "Baroque" is the adjective she borrows from the philosopher Christine Buci-Glucksmann to suggest this alternative aesthetic logic and way of seeing; a visual style that prefers irregularity and extravagance to simplicity, and elevates wonder over intelligibility.[101]

This book, too, is concerned with the ethics of looking and the aesthetics of difference, but it approaches ethics and aesthetics through specific visual encounters. One of the questions addressed here is *how*—under what conditions and by what means—does the grotesque, the horrific, or the ugly become beautiful; the abject, sublime? For Garland-Thomson, artistic representations of disability and disfigurement are valuable because they grant us "permission to stare" and invite "empathy" and "sensitivity."[102] But the possibility of seeing difference differently is not just a matter of representation. Underpinning her account of disability and beauty is an understanding of both as social and dynamic. It is not the artist who creates or reveals beauty; it is the staree who shows people "how to look."[103] In the context of war, disabled and disfigured bodies are burdened with meaning; they become symbols of nationhood and allegories of loss. Although the voices of those who were wounded in the Great War may now be absent—and in most cases unrecoverable—it is beholden on us to imagine them looking back.

CHAPTER 1

The Elusive Portrait

> It would be a mistake to think that we only need to find the right and true images, and that a certain reality will then be conveyed.[1]
> —Judith Butler, *Precarious Life: The Powers of Mourning and Violence*

2008

The war in Afghanistan, "Operation Enduring Freedom," was about to enter its seventh and most violent year yet. President Bush was planning the "quiet surge" that would see the total number of U.S. troops increase to over thirty-five thousand. Coalition deaths and serious injuries had risen exponentially: in 2008 there were 295 military fatalities (roughly half of which were U.S. personnel), and 795 U.S. troops were recorded wounded in action.[2] Meanwhile, on the campaign trail, presidential candidates John McCain, Hillary Clinton, and Barack Obama voiced their opinions on withdrawal from Iraq: McCain arguing for maintaining troop levels; Clinton advocating a full withdrawal; and Obama calling Operation Iraqi Freedom a "massive strategic blunder."[3] That year alone, more than two thousand American servicemen and women returned home from Iraq with serious injuries. Yet the iconic media images were not of the dead and the wounded; they were the bloodless spectacles of "shock and awe" and "precision bombing" and the constant stream of anecdotal reports filed by journalists embedded with Coalition troops.[4]

The Iraq War has been the "most intensively reported war in history," notes Julian Stallabrass in *Memory of Fire: Images of War and the War of*

Images. In World War I, the British government's propaganda bureau appointed one official photographer to each theater of war (including the civilian effort at home) with the exception of the western front, which was deemed important enough to require several photographers.[5] When the invasion of Iraq began in March 2003, the Pentagon authorized up to 750 "embeds."[6] As Stallabrass points out, embedding had the obvious advantage of allowing "largely uncensored access to military operations" while encouraging in reporters "a positive view of what they saw."

> Since many embedded journalists were placed in dangerous circumstances under the protection of the troops, and lived with them for extended periods, this usually fostered a strong identification with their new comrades. They were generally grateful for the access to spectacular stories, admiring of their protectors, and appreciative of the troops' various travails.[7]

By the end of 2006, however, there were only twenty-six journalists embedded with U.S. forces in Iraq: a trend that reflected the escalating costs of the occupation and insurgency (for media organizations as well as the Pentagon) and the fact that exhausted troops, mutilated bodies, and traumatized civilians had become a turnoff to advertisers and politicians alike. Speaking about his own experience of Iraq in 2008, photojournalist Michael Kamber describes a proliferating array of regulations:

> Today in Iraq there's so many things we can't photograph any more. Car bombings and suicide bombings are now off limits, it's actually illegal to photograph those scenes. We can't photograph wounded soldiers without their consent. We can't photograph dead soldiers, coffins of dead soldiers. . . . We can't photograph battle-damage vehicles; we can't photograph hospitals; morgues are off limits now. So pretty much everything that gives evidence that there's a war going on is almost impossible to photograph.[8]

Writing in the *Guardian* the same year, Dan Kennedy, an associate professor of journalism at Northeastern University in Boston, called the photographic record of the war "antiseptic," pointing out that in the post–Vietnam War era it had become "increasingly difficult for journalists to cover war in all its horror."[9] The (by then) four thousand dead Americans—and many thousands more who had been seriously wounded—were off limits to journalists and largely unseen by the public.[10]

One publication stands out against this backdrop of "bloodless and anodyne" reporting.[11] In the summer of 2008 the U.S. Office of the Surgeon General published a collection of case studies of trauma surgery in Iraq and Afghanistan.[12] Each chapter was illustrated with photographs provided by U.S. Army medical officers, most of them taken on personal digital cameras. *War Surgery in Afghanistan and Iraq* is "war without the war story," Sue Halpern observed in the *New York Review of Books*.[13] There is no plot, no characterization, no "good guys" and "bad guys" (although duty is mentioned more than once). Open the book and what you see, close-up and in full color, are the physical consequences of war: for civilians—the casualties here include children—as well as combatants. These include multiple facial wounds impregnated with sand and rocks, 80 percent body burn, traumatic evisceration, and genital soft-tissue trauma. Yet the first image in the book is not of human wreckage; it is a double-page photograph showing the blank expanse of a concrete wall and a sun-bleached road sign, in English and Arabic, pointing the way to Baghdad passenger terminals. There are no figures in this postapocalyptic landscape; just a dusty verge, a few weeds the only sign of life. The following page contains this epigraph:

> It is impossible to convey to you the picture of human misery continually before my eye . . . While I amputated one man's thigh, there lay at one time thirteen, all beseeching to be taken next . . . It was a strange thing to feel my clothes stiff with blood, and my arms powerless with the exertion of using the knife! . . . The view of the field, the gallant sorties, the charges, the individual instances of enterprise and valour recalled to me the sense the world has of victory and Waterloo. But this is transient. A gloomy uncomfortable view of human nature is the inevitable consequence of looking upon the whole as I did—as I was forced to do.

The author of these words was the Scottish anatomist, surgeon, and artist Sir Charles Bell (1774–1842), who in 1815 treated, and drew, injuries sustained in the Battle of Waterloo. Bell's weary evocation of humanity's capacity for destruction is echoed in the afterword, which pairs a photograph of a solitary, unnamed soldier overcome with grief and exhaustion with the famous line from Virgil's *Aeneid*: *sunt lacrimae rerum et mentem mortalia tangunt*—"these are the tears of things, and our mortality cuts to the heart." Military censors apparently tried to prevent the book's commercial release. They needn't have bothered. As a reviewer notes on Amazon, "This book is likely to attract only a small readership who are interested in the different challenges in these conflict areas." Intended for use by military surgeons, the coffee table-sized volume is a compendium of contemporary combat injuries and their treatment. These are pictures you won't see on the evening news, but they are also images that most of us would rather not see.

War Surgery in Afghanistan and Iraq is the degree zero of war representation. What it demonstrates is that the visibility (or not) of war is as much about what we want to, or can bear to, look at as it is about issues of press censorship and journalistic freedom. This chapter considers the ways in which some of the most politically damaging consequences of recent military operations have become visible, with a particular emphasis on the representation of veterans with disabling and disfiguring injuries in the period between President Bush's declaration of the "War on Terror" in 2001 and Barack Obama's inauguration in January 2009. How has the disfigured or disabled body of the war veteran been presented to the American and British public? A number of recurring themes can be identified, the most pervasive being the rhetoric of "heroic individualism" that has characterized the limited portrayal of wounded soldiers in the news media and in documentaries like HBO's acclaimed *Alive Day Memories: Home From Iraq.*[14]

The Theater of War

An "alive day" is a day you almost die. On an empty, blacked-out soundstage in downtown Manhattan in the winter of 2006, the actor and executive producer of *Alive Day Memories*, James Gandolfini, interviewed eight men and two women who survived life-threatening injuries in Iraq. Ranging in age from twenty-one to forty-one, they describe in detail the events that resulted in amputation, brain injury, facial reconstruction, blindness and post-traumatic stress syndrome. All but one of the stories is told in the first person. The exception is former marine sergeant Eddie Ryan, whose cognitive impairment is so severe that his mother speaks for him, holding his hand as she describes the effects that two bullets to the head have had on her child. The testimonies are intercut with home videos and photographs as well as footage taken in Iraq: some of it filmed on vehicle-mounted cameras used in combat missions; some of it taken by embedded American journalists, and some of it released by Iraqi insurgents following similar IED (improvised explosive device) attacks. The interviews were broadcast on HBO between September 9 and 16, 2007: a scheduling decision that underlines the broader commemorative intent of the project as well as its political significance. As Fred Turner notes in his review for the *Journal of American History*, "*Alive Day Memories* brings to the screen a kind of suffering that the George W. Bush administration has worked hard to make invisible."[15]

Gandolfini explains that the idea for the interviews came about during a visit to the Walter Reed Army Medical Center in Washington, D.C.[16] The head of HBO's documentary division, Sheila Nevins, had wanted to make a follow-up to *Baghdad E.R.*, which looked at the Iraq War through the eyes of military medical personnel: this series would focus on some of the men and women whose lives had been saved.[17] Two weeks before filming was due to start, they were told by military officials that Walter Reed was off limits. "There was no explanation why," says Nevins, but the authorities must have suspected an antiwar agenda (Nevins is open about her personal opposition to America's role in Iraq).[18] Working independently, she managed to track down veterans who had been discharged from Walter Reed; the producers hired a small performance space, and the interviews went ahead. The minimal set (a few chairs and a strip of colored stage lights) adds a theatrical dimension to the performances, which seem at times like dramatic monologues. Gandolfini's demeanor is respectful to the point of self-effacement: having asked a question he leans back into the shadows and listens. "He didn't want the cameras on him," commented former marine corporal Jake Schick.[19] The respect is clearly mutual. In an interview with the *New York Times*, John Jones, a former marine staff sergeant, recalls watching DVDs of *The Sopranos* projected onto a bathroom wall in Iraq. Tony Soprano and his gang were their role models, he says: "We'd talk about the godfather (the commanding officer) and the lieutenant would tell us to go out and put a hit on a guy."[20] In the stage interviews violence is something perpetrated by Iraqis—not Americans—and Tony Soprano has been sublimated into an altogether gentler alter ego (although Gandolfini admits in an interview that watching video footage of insurgent attacks "makes you want to pick up a gun and kill somebody").[21]

In its restrained theatricality and emotive power, *Alive Day Memories* couldn't be more different from *War Surgery in Afghanistan and Iraq*. There are similarities, though: not least of all the strange confluence of spectacles that give us our theaters of war, surgery and drama: a set of associations not lost on Nevins.[22] The English word "theater" comes from the Greek θέατρον (*théatron*, "a place for viewing"), an etymology that should remind us that medicine and war have always involved an element (variously enjoyed and disapproved) of the spectacular. The other common element is the therapeutic discourse that has come to define the popular response to unpopular wars in the twentieth and twenty-first centuries. Already apparent in World War I, the rhetoric of "mending" broken soldiers—or "renovating" damaged faces—has transformed the idea and image of sacrifice.[23] No longer the beautiful death of the classical tradition—a fantasy that was finally put to rest on the battlefields of the Great War—modern sacrifice follows a medical paradigm of injury, treatment, and rehabilitation: this is the journey that Gandolfini's interviewees take us on, although for all of them, recovery is partial and ongoing.

Turner locates the emergence of the therapeutic idiom in the post–Vietnam War era and points out that the tendency to focus on individual suffering and courage—usually the suffering and courage of individual Americans—has several effects. Most problematically, it can serve (deliberately or not) to depoliticize war and conflict. *Alive Day Memories,* he observes, "never asks how or why America came to Iraq in the first place, or why U.S. troops remain there." Nor does it extend the discourse of suffering to the Iraqis, who appear as "faceless voices in insurgent videos or as blasted corpses in post-attack snapshots." Distanced from its historical and political contexts, combat is seen "as individual, even private experience."[24]

Gandolfini's position was that the film had no political point of view. When the news anchor Brian Williams raised the issue on *NBC Nightly News* a few days before the HBO premiere, Gandolfini replied: "I wanted to hear what they [the veterans] had to say. And I think sometimes, when something is political, half of the people will shut down immediately and not listen."[25] The real subject of the film is not the war in Iraq and its consequences: it is "honor, duty, loyalty to your country."[26] And the appropriate response to such profound acts of patriotism is not political, the film implies, it is emotional (and also medical: a point to which we shall return).[27] Dawn Halfaker, whose right arm and shoulder were amputated following a grenade attack, wonders if her child—if she ever has one—will love her as she is. Gandolfini waits in silence as her face clouds with emotion. "What were you thinking just then?" he asks gently. "I won't be able to pick up my son or daughter with two arms and hold them," she replies.

It is impossible not to be moved by what Halfaker and the other interviewees describe: to admire their fortitude, conviction, and honesty. But we also need to ask how their stories shape our understanding of war and patriotism. Whether tragic or celebratory, the discursive and visual "frames of war" (to borrow Judith Butler's phrase) serve to "organize visual experience" and mobilize affect.[28] To a significant extent, they determine what we see and what we feel. The very concept of humanity—damaged or triumphant—has become an ideological battleground in which representations themselves are "modes of military conduct."[29] For Butler, however, framing is always provisional. Commenting on the photographs that sparked the 2004 Abu Ghraib scandal, she questions Susan Sontag's assertion that photographs of suffering and atrocity are not in themselves meaningful; that our understanding of them depends entirely on external factors such as captions, accompanying text, and the circumstances in which we encounter the image.[30]

While Butler does not deny that photographs of war can be reframed and reinterpreted—or that they mean different things in different contexts—she insists on the potential of images themselves to create *new* contexts, and this is where her analysis departs most decisively from Sontag's. The state can make every effort to regulate the visual representation of war by embedding journalists within military units and placing restrictions on what the media can print or broadcast, but ultimately every attempt to dictate what we should see and feel is temporary. Images like those taken at Abu Ghraib—that confound or "break out" of the prevailing frames of war—have the potential to disturb the "quotidian acceptance" of violence and replace it with outrage. Nowhere is this slippage of meaning more evident than on the Internet, where the circulation and interpretation of images is so difficult to limit or direct. Butler's point is not just that we need a more democratic and ethical news media, or more truthful images of war. Her concern is to elucidate (or as she puts it, to "frame") the very frames that make violence possible:

> To learn to see the frame that blinds us to what we see is no easy matter. *And if there is a crucial role for visual culture during times of war it is precisely to thematize the forcible frame*, the one that conducts the dehumanizing norm, that restricts what is perceivable, and indeed, what can be.[31]

Dora Apel's *War Culture and the Contest of Images* (2012) can be read as a response to this call. Focusing on representations of war in the United States and the Middle East since 9/11, Apel argues that two discourses have dominated—one might say framed—artists' and photographers' responses to war (her case studies range from Nina Berman to Banksy). The first is the discourse of "heroic individualism," which "looks for signs of healing, hope, and hardiness as evidence that the free individual can transcend the most oppressive circumstances."[32] The counternarrative focuses on "the responsibility of the state, which is held accountable for the arrested development and truncated lives of the soldiers whom it uses up and spits out."[33] These sound like mutually exclusive alternatives—one serving to legitimize militarism; the other manifestly antiwar—but in reality they can coexist. *Alive Day Memories* is one such example. Although it has all the features of heroic individualism, the rhetoric of "overcoming" (the individual's overcoming of pain, injury, disability, stigma) is never entirely convincing because it feels like a necessary fiction, born of the survivor's need—and ours—to believe that suffering *can* be transcended, whether through medical intervention, religious faith, love and friendship, or patriotism.

In keeping with Butler's *Frames of War*, one of the themes of Apel's book is the excess and instability of meaning in documentary photographs of war: an idea that she illustrates with Timothy Greenfield-Sanders's portrait of Dawn Halfaker (figure 2). A celebrity photographer best known for his contributions to *Vanity Fair*, Greenfield-Sanders was commissioned by HBO to produce the thirteen portraits that appeared in the publicity for the documentary, on billboards and, through September 2007, as blowups displayed in the street-level windows of the Donnell Library across from MOMA in New York (where a free screening of the film was held). Discussing Greenfield-Sanders's portraits in *Art in America*, Marcia Vetrocq notes the photographer's trademark monochrome background and format.[34] Close-up or full figure, the subjects fill their frames and face us directly. "We *know* that his portraits are posed," Vetrocq continues. "We *know* that his particular, direct mode of address democratically imparts a quotient of glamour to all his subjects."[35] At the edge of each print, the border of the photographic negative is just visible. Greenfield-Sanders conjures with the conventions of photographic portraiture while drawing attention to the artifice of those conventions.

Halfaker's luminous portrait is the photographer's favorite, although he initially felt uncomfortable suggesting the pose we see in the final image.[36] Dressed casually in jeans and a light sweater and seen from the thighs up, she holds her artificial right arm so that it curves across her torso from breast to hip. Unlike the mechanical prostheses worn by the other veterans in the series, it is the naturalism of Halfaker's arm that is shocking in this image. The evident weight of the limb, its realistic complexion (complete with freckles), and the addition of a silver wrist-

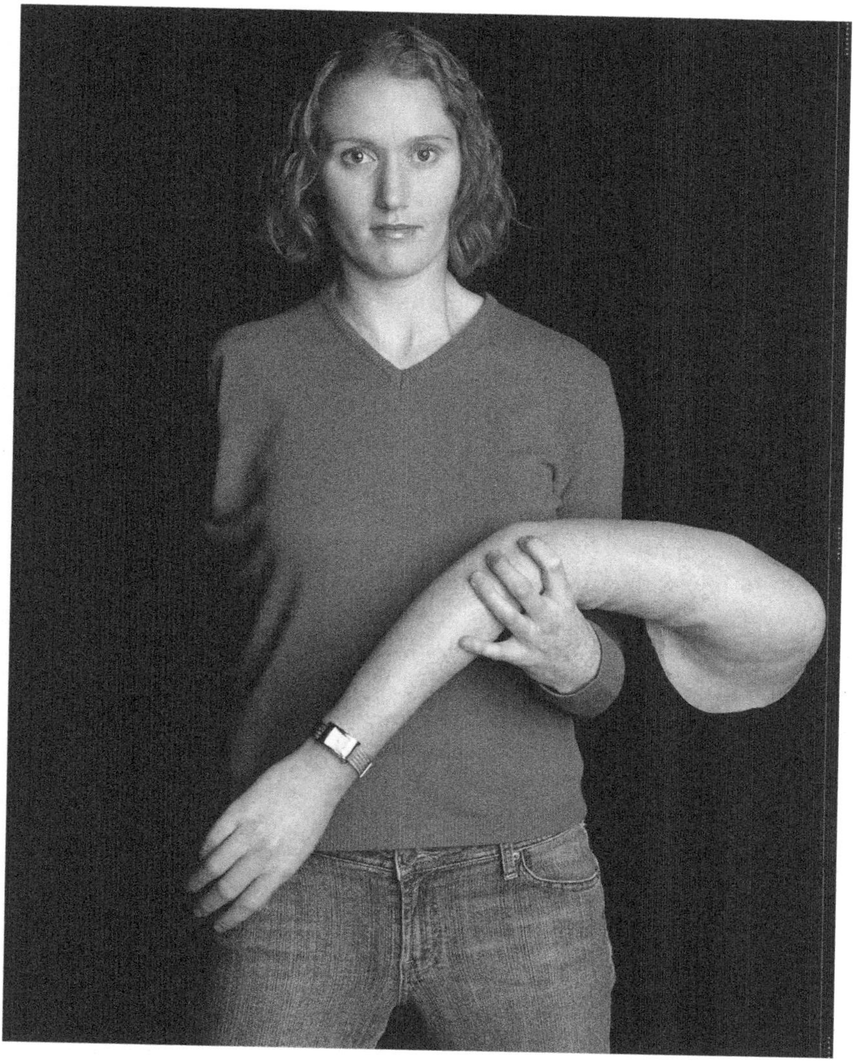

Fig. 2. Timothy Greenfield-Sanders, *Dawn Halfaker,* 2006, digital pigment print, 40 × 30 inches. (© Timothy Greenfield-Sanders, courtesy of the photographer.)

watch create the illusion of an actual arm and shoulder detached and rotated. Of the soldiers and marines interviewed for *Alive Day Memories,* Dawn Halfaker is the only one who expresses any real concern about her changed appearance. At Walter Reed she refused to wear the prosthetics they gave her. "I don't want to look like a robot," she told them, "and I don't want to wear a frickin' hook."[37] Her determination comes across in the portrait, but as Apel argues, "the sense of heroic agency" is unsettled by the poignancy of the watch, by the almost perfect arm (that cannot hold a child), and ultimately by the moments of doubt and disillusionment Halfaker betrays in the telling of her story.[38]

We might conclude, with Apel, that images of the war-damaged body are inherently unpredictable: you can press them into the service of one story (patriotism or human resilience, for example), but they always threaten to reveal another. The rest of this chapter looks closely at the work of two contemporary photographers who have sought more explicitly than Greenfield-Sanders to challenge the ideology of heroic individualism. To the extent that they seek to give abstract statistics a human face, Nina Berman (b. 1960, New York City) and Stuart Griffiths (b. Manchester, 1972) share Greenfield-Sanders's aims, but they differ profoundly in their awareness of the social and psychological ramifications of violence. Asked during a talk at the 2010 Whitney Biennial why she was initially drawn to war photography, Berman described a trip to Vietnam in 1987 with a group of Vietnam vets. She realized that for them "the war hadn't stopped."[39] The news media's fetishistic obsession with the violence of combat obscures both the ongoing effects of war and its cultural preconditions (the subject of a more recent project by Berman documenting military training exercises and large-scale simulations).[40] Elaborating further on her decision to focus on the veterans returning from Iraq, she says:

> I think that part of our lack of understanding of war is that there is so much imagery of that combat moment and very little imagery of the years and years, and the ripple effects after. . . . And as there were no images of wounded Americans or dead Americans, I thought that was something that I could do.[41]

Berman started making portraits of Iraq veterans in 2003, scouring local newspapers online for information about wounded heroes returning home. The series chronicles the stories of nineteen men and one woman through recorded interviews and photographs taken with a six-by-six Hasselblad.[42] The photographs, along with printed excerpts from the interviews, were published in 2004 as *Purple Hearts: Back from Iraq*. Many of the portraits were taken at the soldiers' homes; others show the long process of rehabilitation at Brooke Army Medical Center in Texas and Walter Reed Military Hospital in Washington, D.C. (figures 3 and 4). In his introduction to the book, the author Verlyn Klinkenborg writes: "It's hard to say just when the word 'hero' went bankrupt."

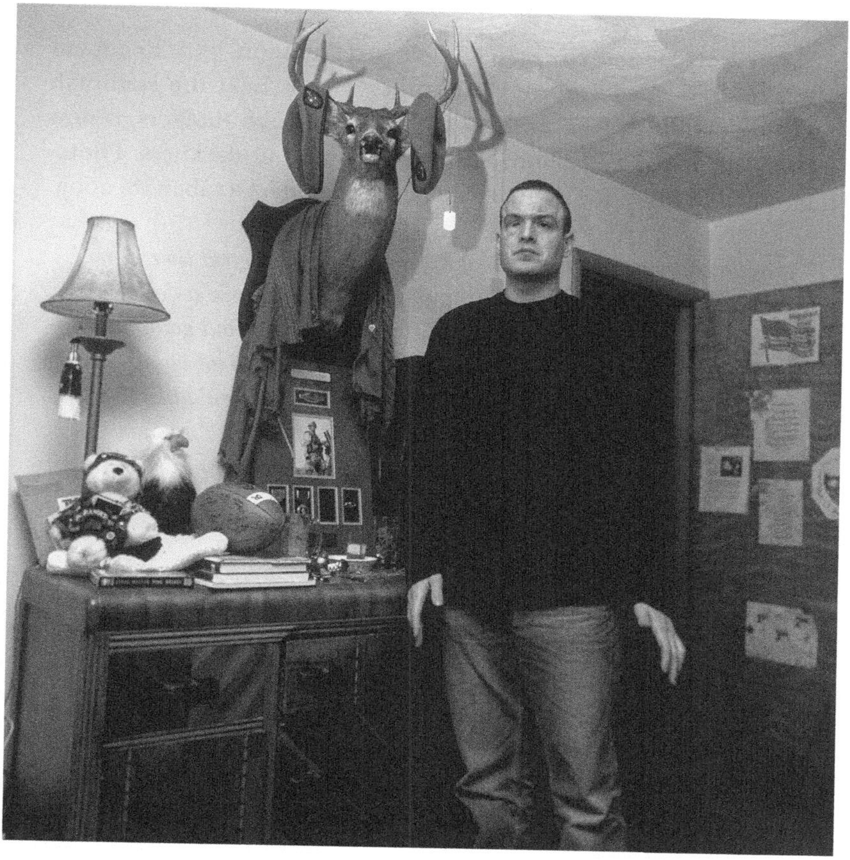

Fig. 3. Nina Berman, *Purple Hearts*, 2004, pigment print, 28 inches square. Jeremy Feldbusch, photographed at his home in Blairsville, Pennsylvania, 2003. (© Photo by Nina Berman / NOOR.)

No one has the right to say that these soldiers are not heroes. But I also suspect that few people understand the contemporary hollowness of that word better than they do. To a soldier coming home from war, the word "hero" looks surprisingly like a gesture of incomprehension, especially in our time when the word is on everyone's lips. It measures the appalling gap between civilians and soldiers, the inexplicable difference between war and peace.[43]

Stuart Griffiths was living in a hostel for homeless ex-servicemen in East London when he decided to start documenting the lives of his fellow residents. A former soldier in the British Army's Parachute Regiment, he had spent five years in Northern Ireland in the late 1980s and early

Sgt. Jeremy Feldbusch, 24, a Ranger, 3rd Battalion, 75th Regiment was injured April 3, during an artillery attack near the Hadithah Dam. Feldbusch, who was first in his class of 228 Rangers, is now brain damaged and blind. He sees nothing but darkness. Photographed in his home in Blairsville, Pennsylvania, October 18, 2003.

I graduated from the University of Pittsburgh. I had a great time there. I was a biology major. At one point in my life, I wanted to be a doctor.

Even while I was going through college, I thought about going into the military. And when I was done, it was brought up to me again, about going into the army, and I thought, you know what, I would like to do that. There were lots of other things I could have done but I was just like, you know, I want to do that, and I talked to recruiters around here, I knew the commander of the recruiting station and he was trying to get me signed.

Before I went, I knew about the Middle East as much as I needed to. But it didn't make a difference. I wasn't fighting a political war with them anyway. That was already taken care of. It was a new kind of war that was going to be fought, so that was where I was stepping in.

That's about it. I don't have any regrets. I had some fun over there. I don't want to talk about the military anymore.

Fig. 4. "I knew about the Middle East as much as I needed to." (Facing text page in *Purple Hearts*.)

1990s, first as a rifleman and then as a photographer with his unit's intelligence section. His snapshots from that period—taken on a instamatic camera—are the visual equivalent of a diary, capturing the mundane details of army life, but also its "underlying tension."[44] Griffiths went on to complete a degree in photography at the University of Brighton, drifted in and out of menial jobs, and ended up, in 2000, sleeping rough in London while trying to get work as paparazzi photographer. New Belvedere House in Stepney, East London, became his home for almost a year, although he describes it as "one of the most lonesome places on earth."[45] At the time, there were about one hundred ex-service personnel living there, many of whom were coping with physical or psychological trauma in addition to alcohol or drug addiction.

In 2003 Griffiths returned to New Belvedere House because he "thought the story of the hostel needed to be told" as "a kind of warning."[46] Before long he was taking photographs of veterans returning from Iraq and Afghanistan whose careers had come to an abrupt end in rehabilitation centers, in halfway houses, or on the streets. Their stories—and Griffiths's own—are told in *Isolation*, a documentary feature by Luke Seomore and Joseph Bull that premiered at the Edinburgh International Film Festival in 2009. With its impressionistic cinematography and a soundtrack that one reviewer described as "the closest thing I've experienced in a film to undergoing a breakdown,"[47] *Isolation* is very much in the "artistic" documentary tradition. Seomore explains that they wanted to capture the quality of Griffiths's photography in film, and to make the conversations between Griffiths and the other ex-soldiers as intimate as possible.[48]

War and the Photographic Portrait

Photographic portraiture has become a primary means of framing war in contemporary Western culture. It is through the portrait (and its textual equivalent, the biography) that we have come to experience—to *feel*—the human dimension of violent conflict. This is particularly true of professional photojournalism, which relies above all on the emotional legibility and expressiveness of the face.[49] What's more, the discourses identified by Apel—heroic individualism and state responsibility—rely on the evidentiary claims of both photography (as documentary record) and portraiture (as a visible indicator of fortitude or trauma). These are not just literary tropes or war stories that conform to narrative conventions: they are visual, embodied discourses, and more specifically, constellations of ideas and emotions that seem to require a face. Not every image of a face is a portrait, however, and portraiture does not always require facial likeness: Picasso's cubist portraits don't look much like their subjects—not in a mimetic sense—and contemporary portraiture often disrupts the conventional association between facial appearance and identity.[50] What, then, does it mean to "put a face" to suffering and violence?[51] And what are the effects (and limits) of traditional portraiture when the face itself has been transformed by war?

In *Precarious Life: The Powers of Mourning and Violence* Judith Butler questions the assumption that representation bestows humanity on the otherwise faceless, anonymous statistics of war. Faces in the media, she points out, can, and often do, personify evil, or liberation, or terror. The now iconic faces of Yasser Arafat, Saddam Hussein, and Osama bin Laden are a case in point. Variations on a common theme—the media "portrait of evil"—they were used to personify deception (Arafat), tyranny (Hussein), and terror (bin Laden).[52] This is the human face "in its deformity and extremity," writes Butler. It is both a caution and an explanation, as generic and didactic as the faces of saints.

In much the same way, the faces of "liberated" (unveiled) Afghan women serve as emblems of "American cultural progress,"[53] and the faces of children symbolize innocence and the exquisite fragility of life. Photojournalism exploits the human face's capacity to convey a sense of the individual while at the same time signifying a generic type, attribute, or emotion: the face of suffering, the face of evil. Not surprisingly, many artists and photographers have sought to distance themselves from such clichés. If the human face of war is ubiquitous in the news media and on television, it is often entirely absent from museums and art galleries. Some of the most compelling contemporary photographs of war are devoid of human subject matter, dwelling instead on the postapocalyptic aftermath of conflict: urban wastelands, architectural ruins, depopulated villages, and the surreal topography of battle-scarred landscapes or mass graves. One of the most successful proponents of this subgenre of the "military sublime," Simon Norfolk, has said that he prefers taking pictures of landscapes because "people gobble up the photograph. They become what the photograph *is*." If he does include people, "It's usually because they represent an idea."[54]

Norfolk's large-format photographs of postinvasion Baghdad were shown alongside work by Paul Seawright, Adam Broomberg, and Oliver Chanarin at the 2008 Brighton Photo Biennial in a themed exhibition, "The Sublime Image of Destruction." Stallabrass (the Biennial's curator) and Norfolk initially wanted to include an enlarged print of a seriously injured Iraqi child in Zafaraniah Hospital, Baghdad. "[We] wanted to show the image because it frankly described the consequences of the war," Stallabrass recalls.[55] Norfolk had been urged to take the photograph by the Iraqis who were present at the scene: in it we see eighteen-month-old Zainab Tharmar, her small face smeared with blood, lying with her eyes closed on a brightly patterned bedspread (figure 5). A sheet of white gauze placed lightly over her soiled yellow dress is the only sign of medical intervention. He must have leaned over the bed to get close enough: you can almost touch the pink fleece of the blanket and feel the child's downy hair.

That the portrait of Zainab Tharmar "puts a face" to the horrors

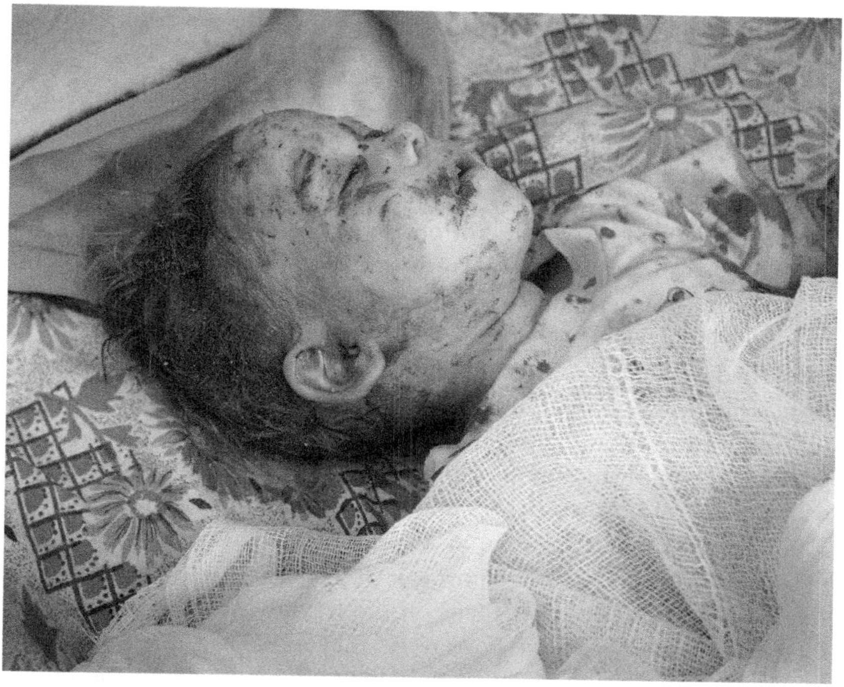

Fig. 5. Simon Norfolk, 18-month-old Zainab Tharmar, seriously wounded by an American-controlled explosion of Iraqi missiles. Many facts about this incident are disputed. Zafaraniah Hospital, Baghdad, April 26, 2003. (© Simon Norfolk / INSTITUTE.)

of war is unarguable, but placed alongside images of sublime destruction, the photograph raised a number of intractable questions for Stallabrass and the curators at Brighton's De La Warr Pavilion: "How did the image, with its focus on the face of an individual, fit with the more general scenes of ruination in the exhibition? What did the inflation of size do to its meaning as the depiction of an individual? Had the child survived (viewers would surely want to know)?" In the end, they decided not to use the print on the grounds that to do so would be to reduce Zainab Tharmar "to an icon of the general"—an object lesson on the consequences of war. This is a dilemma for anyone engaged with the representation of war: "that the cruelties depicted are typical, and that they happen to individuals."[56] For Sarah James, who collaborated with Stallabrass on *Memory of Fire*, Norfolk's photograph of Zainab Tharmar does something else. It shows what is absent from the sublime image of destruction. "The contemplative sublime cannot accommodate flesh, bodies or selves," she writes: "how then can it produce empathy, or awareness of fellow suffering?"[57]

The Management of Spoiled Identity

Empathy is not a prerequisite for portraiture, at least not as it has traditionally been understood. The word "portrait," notes Ludmilla Jordanova, "has an air of formality to it; it conjures up both a pose, for a specific purpose, and a maker, someone who is more than a friend, a relation or casual acquaintance."[58] A portrait is more than a snapshot, and different from a medical photograph, in part because it bestows authority on the subject portrayed (and also implicitly on the maker).[59] Historically, the portrait—certainly the commissioned portrait—has been a form of physical capital, as Bourdieu defines it: an investment in one's public face.[60] The image of Zainab Tharmar and the photographs of veterans by Berman and Griffiths are more equivocal. Unlike Greenfield-Sanders's *Alive Day Memories* portraits, they focus on the fragility of subjectivity; rather than "consolidating the self portrayed," they reveal its vulnerability.[61]

In all of the examples discussed above the authority of the photographic subject is precarious. Berman and Griffiths do not portray injured veterans as victims, but nor are they "survivors" in the popular sense of the term. Their images don't make an overt appeal to a common humanity (like humanitarian portraits of suffering): they are, rather, portraits of irrevocably damaged humanity. Reviewing *Marine Wedding* for the *New York Times*, Holland Cotter describes Tyler Ziegel's expression, as he looks at his bride, as "hard to read: his dead-white face is all but featureless, with no nose and no chin, as blank as a pullover mask." Despite winning the World Press Photo Contest for portraiture, the photograph challenges the premise of the traditional portrait: that the face can be relied upon as an index of identity and emotion (figure 1). Like Berman's earlier project *Purple Hearts, Marine Wedding* focuses on the homecoming: the protracted and difficult—perhaps ultimately impossible—transition from the military to civilian life, from able-bodied soldier or marine to disabled veteran. Berman thinks it unlikely that *People* magazine had seen a picture of Ziegel when they approached her with the commission. It was supposed to be a happy story: wounded war hero, high school sweethearts, fairy-tale wedding. When she first met Ziegel, she was shocked at the extent of his injuries. "I've seen lots of wounded people before," she comments in an interview with Richard Bradley, "but he was probably the worst-looking, and also the least expressive." She wondered why, "after all this time," *People* had picked someone who was "going to be so physically a turnoff."[62]

Although Ziegel was possibly "the least self-conscious person [she had] ever met," it was obvious that "part of the story had to be how people look at him"—and to that extent *Marine Wedding* is about the stigma of disability and disfigurement as Erving Goffman describes it, "within a particular social interaction." By the time Goffman was writing *Stigma: Notes on the Management of Spoiled Identity* in the early 1960s, there was already a substantial literature on the subject in social psychology and sociology. The term itself, however, has a much longer history. In the original Greek, the verb "stigmatize" meant quite literally to mark or brand with a hot iron. Such a stigma would identify the bearer as a criminal, a slave, or a traitor.[63] Adapted by early Christians, the word came to denote "bodily signs of holy grace that took the form of eruptive blossoms on the skin," but the idea that one could be "marked" by God coexisted with a proto-medical understanding of stigma as a symptom of physical or moral disorder.[64] Even today, this indexical logic persists. In Ziegel's case, we are likely to read his scars as the indication (in Charles Sanders Peirce's terms) of an invisible condition: proof not of God's grace or of human wickedness, but of the traumatizing and dehumanizing effects of war.[65]

Goffman's contribution was to illuminate the relational nature of stigma. It is not the case, he argues, that certain conditions or characteristics are stigmatizing in themselves. There *is* no indelible mark. Rather, "normal" and "stigmatized" are shifting perspectives that depend on one's expectations of others within a particular context.[66] He gives the example of a professional criminal who fears being seen entering his local public library and always checks over his shoulder. A love of books is considered perfectly normal in some circles and stigmatizing in others. Both normality and stigma are "a special kind of relationship between attribute [in this case "bookishness"] and stereotype ["middle-class boy" or "professional criminal"]."[67]

The same comparison of attribute to stereotype turns physical difference into a deviation from an imagined norm: deformity or disability.[68] "We tend to impute a wide range of imperfections on the basis of the original one," Goffman explains, "and at the same time to impute some desirable but undesired attributes, often of a supernatural cast."[69] The first of these observations can be illustrated by a list of synonyms for "blind" posted on Disability Culture Watch, a blog created by writer and disability arts advocate Simi Linton.[70] They include "ignorant," "imperceptive," "insensitive," "irrational," "oblivious," "obtuse," "random," "rash," "unaware," "unconscious," "uncontrolled," "unknowing," "unplanned," and "violent." "These meanings," observes Linton, "lurk under the surface when the word 'blind' is used whether on its own, or in pairings, in such phrases as 'blind passion,' 'blind rage,' 'blind justice,' 'blind drunk' and 'blind faith.'" On the other hand, blindness is often associated with "inner sight" (the blind prophet or "seer"). Ugliness, too, is implicated in this schema, either as a symptomatic "imperfection" or (much less often) as a physical flaw that signifies inner beauty. This ambivalence is a characteristic of all three types of stigma identified by Goffman: physical deformities, perceived "blemishes of individual character," and "the tribal stigma of race, nation and religion."[71]

One could ask whether Goffman's account of stigma is relevant to visual representations of difference. I think it is, for two reasons. First, Goffman was concerned fundamentally with the cultural construction and social negotiation of stigma. Stereotypes and attributes *are* representations, and visual culture is arguably one of the primary sites of stigmatization. Second, his attention to the intersubjective dynamics of stigma finds an intriguing parallel in the portraits we have been looking at. Art clearly has the potential to reveal the "structural preconditions of stigma," to show that ugliness—like beauty—is negotiated and contingent. Often these negotiations happen prior to or during the making of an image. Berman was aware, for example, that the lighting of the shots was crucial, and wanted to make sure she "didn't make [Ty] look gruesome."[72] Furthermore, some of the photographs take the gaze—or its absence—as their subject. The child in the candy store (figure 6) stares with undisguised amazement at Ty's face: her awareness of his difference is a precondition for stigma, but as yet without moral judgment or "interaction-uneasiness," to use Goffman's term.[73] This is the only image in the series to show someone looking directly at Ziegel, and the lack of visual engagement—especially between Ty and Renee—reinforces the sense of his otherness and her withdrawal.

Griffiths's photographs further complicate the idea that portraiture is a type of likeness that "bestows authority." The veterans he met through New Belvedere House were socially and politically invisible: they literally had no public face. Their lives were—and in many cases still are—"lived behind closed doors."[74] Like Berman, Griffiths had to sidestep the official channels in order to pursue his project independently, and he is openly critical of the Ministry of Defence's attempts to manage the pub-

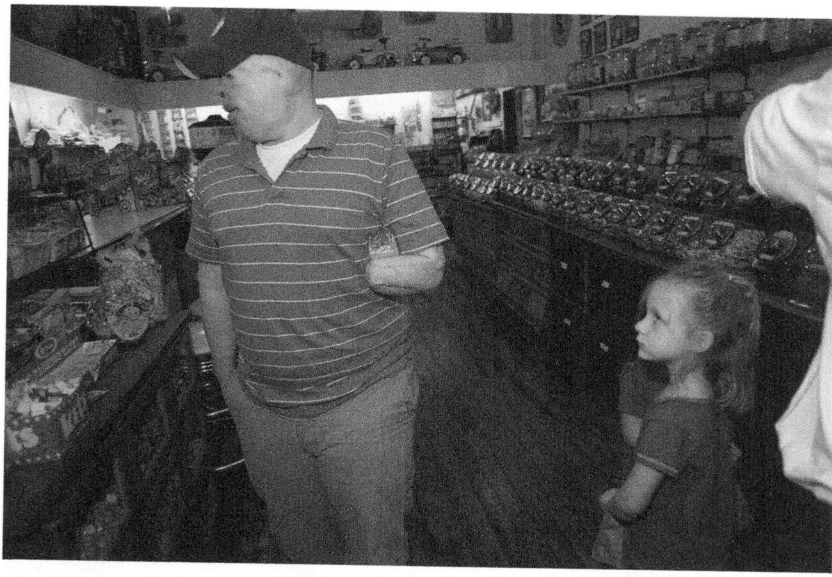

Fig. 6. Nina Berman, *Marine Wedding*, 2006. (© Photo by Nina Berman / NOOR.)

lic image of the armed forces. Refusing to toe the line has had several consequences, the most apparent being the gender and socioeconomic profile of his photographic subjects. With few exceptions (a female medical officer agreed to be interviewed for *Isolation*) they have been young men; most have working-class backgrounds; and none have had high-ranking military careers.[75] A 2008 study of risk factors for PTSD in British armed forces personnel found that "post-traumatic stress symptoms were associated with lower rank, being unmarried, having low educational attainment and a history of childhood adversity."[76] I am not aware of any studies specifically linking PTSD with homelessness, but it is hardly surprising that the same set of circumstances surfaces in Griffiths's interviews with homeless veterans. The one officer he managed to make contact with "got cold feet and contacted the MoD."[77] Griffiths was asked in for an interview and decided against it. On another occasion he was commissioned by *GQ* to do a piece on the military rehabilitation unit at Headley Court in Surrey. On reflection, those photographs are "more institutional, more controlled" than the others: there was no opportunity to interview the patients, and the shoot was stage managed.[78]

Griffiths is ambivalent about the term "portraiture" when applied

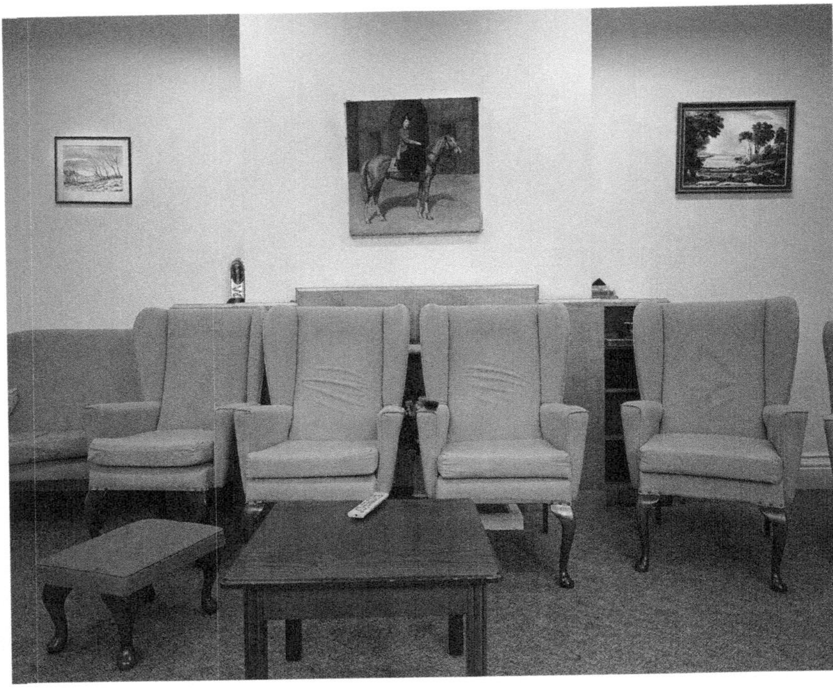

Fig. 7. Stuart Griffiths, Television Room, Combat Stress Rehabilitation Centre, Leatherhead, Surrey, 2006. (© Stuart Griffiths Photographs.)

to his work.[79] In a gallery, the photographs are installed as large-format prints, framed and wall-mounted as single images, in pairs or triptychs, or as groups arranged in irregular columns and rows.[80] Although connections are hinted at, there are no explanatory panels, and the places and people in the photographs are not identified. The biographical content of the exhibition relates to Griffiths himself: his snapshots and doodles of army life; his letters home. Even the title of the show—*Closer*—suggests the photographer's presence. It is his journey we piece together through the lives of others. In a further departure from the conventions of portraiture, several of the figures are seen from behind, or not at all (figure 7). One row of photographs depicts what appears to be a vacated squat from multiple vantage points, its squalid contents visible in forensic detail: cans of Stella, paper Pepsi cups, fag ends and matches, a bloodstained mattress, and, to one side, a patch of vomit on the floor (figure 8). Incongruously, a blue shirt hangs from an otherwise empty wardrobe. A single image on the opposite wall frames a stretch of empty road after rain (figure 9). In the gutter a splash of blood spreads out into a pool of

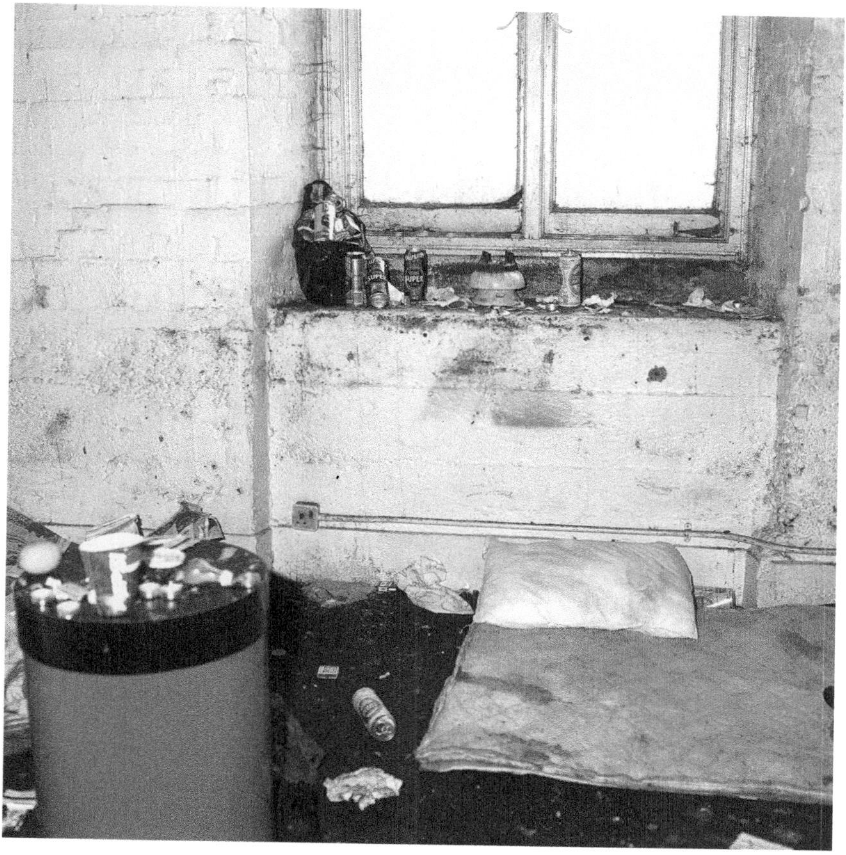

Fig. 8. Stuart Griffiths, Homeless Squat, Kings Cross, London, 2004. (© Stuart Griffiths Photographs.)

dirty water. In a separate triptych of portraits, we see a man with a head injury, the blood still fresh; a pair of legs from the knees down, one badly scarred, the other a mechanical prosthesis; and the disfigured face of a second man (figure 10).

We are invited to speculate about the chains of coincidence that bind these characters, places, and events together. In interviews Griffiths fills in the gaps: in this instance, the injured man is Jason, an ex-soldier living in the veterans' hospital. Stuart had gone with him to the squat in Kings Cross, where Jason's friends supposedly lived, but a man came after them with an iron bar. Jason was beaten and left for dead; Stuart attempted to stop the bleeding while waiting for the ambulance to arrive. Because he had his camera with him, he took an injury claim photograph (something

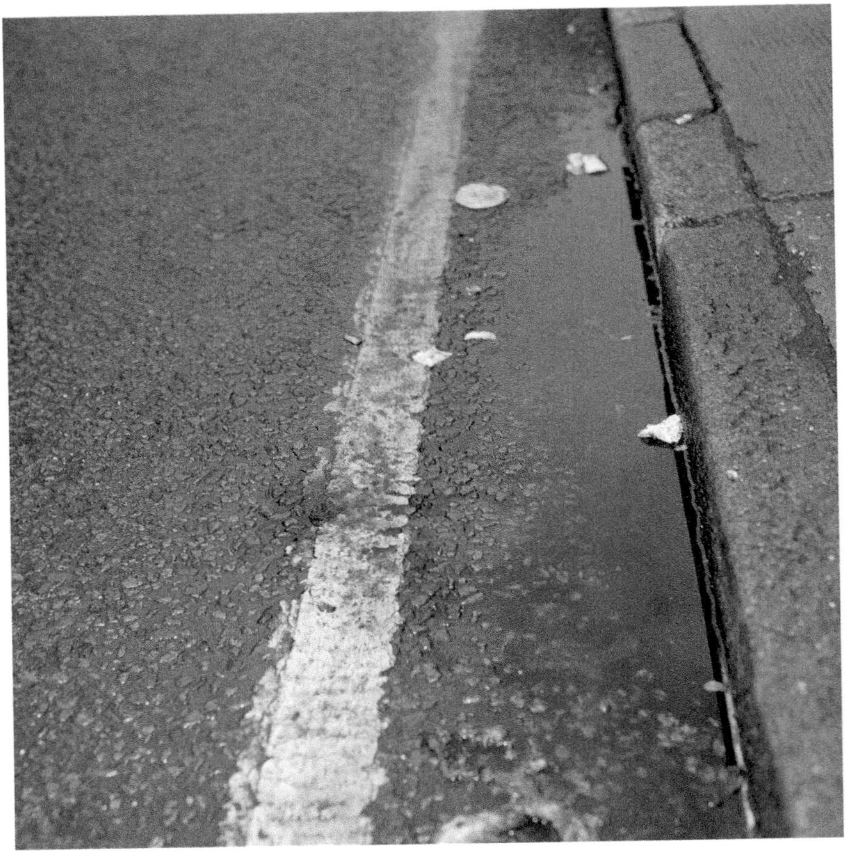

Fig. 9. Stuart Griffiths, Veteran's Blood (moments after being hit in the head with an iron bar), Whitechapel, East London, 2005. (© Stuart Griffiths Photographs.)

he had experience of in Northern Ireland). Shown in a gallery, the image is removed from these circumstances, but even so it serves as a reminder that portraiture is only tenuously distinguished from other kinds of likenesses, including criminal, forensic, and medical photographs.

Griffiths sees his work as a form of "visual protest," an agenda that many (though not all) of the veterans he has photographed share.[81] In keeping with this aim—which is even more apparent in Berman's *Purple Hearts* portraits—the disfigured body of the veteran becomes an accusation rather than a badge of honor or a difficulty to be overcome. Significantly, Griffiths makes no distinction between physical and psychological damage.[82] The men and women in his photographs may bear

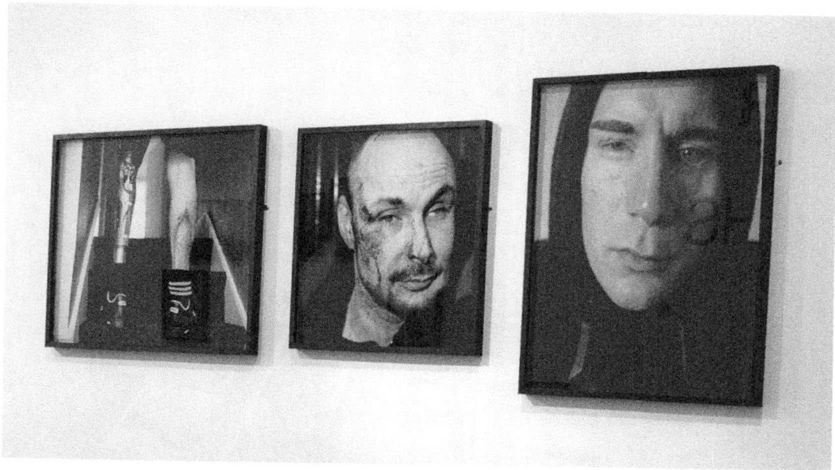

Fig. 10. Stuart Griffiths, Installation of *Closer* at *Moose on the Loose Biennale*, London College of Communication, 2013. (© Stuart Griffiths Photographs.)

visible scars—or not—but the real subject of his work is war's disfiguring effect on the anatomy of society. At times, however, the visual rhetoric of protest—and the irrevocable *otherness* of the war-damaged body—come up against the honorific imperative of portraiture as Allan Sekula describes it in "The Body and the Archive." As discussed in the introduction, nineteenth-century portrait photography evolved from two distinct forms of visual practice: painted portraits (which Sekula defines as "the ceremonial presentation of the bourgeois self") and medical and anatomical illustration (which abstracted the body from the self and presented it as an object of scientific knowledge). With his background in both military *and* celebrity photography, Griffiths seems intuitively aware of these different conventions, and the fact that honorific portrait photography must repress its other (the medical image, injury claim photograph, or ID portrait) in order to perform its ceremonial magic.

When these modalities of portraiture coexist the effect is disturbing. One triptych includes seventeen surgical case photographs placed on a circular dining table and shot from above (figure 11). Although several of the images show the subject's face, it is so lacerated and swollen that identification is impossible. Nor is there any suggestion of a therapeutic narrative: the images are evidence of injury, not recovery. If anything, they suggest Foucault's "anatomical perception"—the modern clinical gaze as an abstraction of the body (or relevant body part) from the person.[83] Blackened nails, punctured and discolored skin, a mass of tubes:

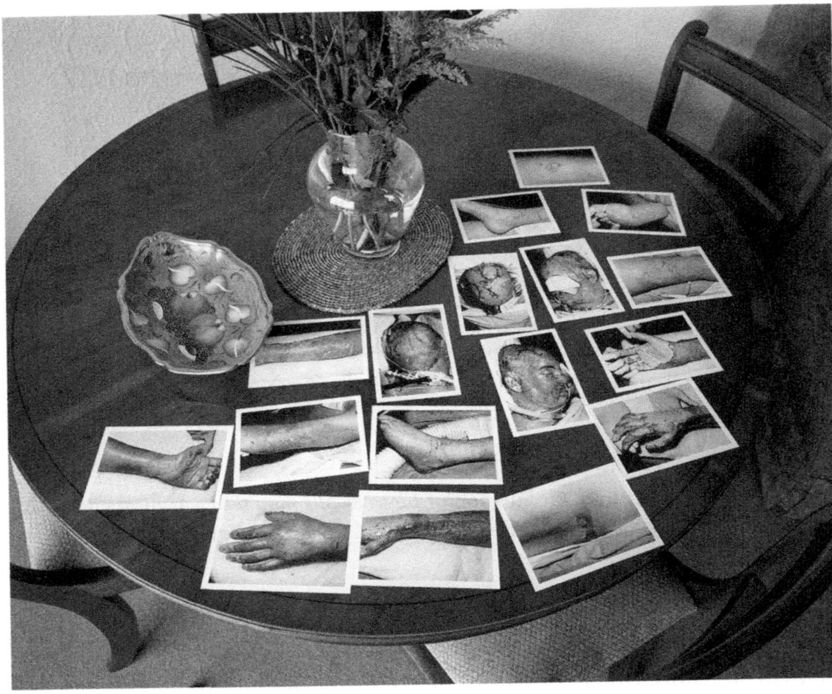

Fig. 11. Stuart Griffiths, Medical photographs of a British soldier who was injured three days into the war in Iraq by friendly fire, Stamford, Lincolnshire, 2006. (© Stuart Griffiths Photographs.)

these are images whose rightful place is the hospital file or medical archive: not a dining room table where they compete for space with a vase of flowers and a pretty fruit bowl. It seems impossible that these realities should coexist, the domestic and the clinical, past trauma and mundane present.

Even when medical photography is not explicitly referenced, however, the tension between protest (aligned here with documentary realism) and portraiture (as an honorific genre) is apparent. Put simply: most of these are photographs you wouldn't want in a family album or on the mantelpiece. To be sure, many of Griffiths's images convey dignity, pride, or defiance, but they also—emphatically—present evidence of suffering, stigma, and neglect. The photographs of Martyn Compton—a torchbearer for the London 2012 Olympics—are particularly interesting in this regard, because Compton's story received so much press coverage in the UK. A lance corporal in the Household Cavalry, Compton sus-

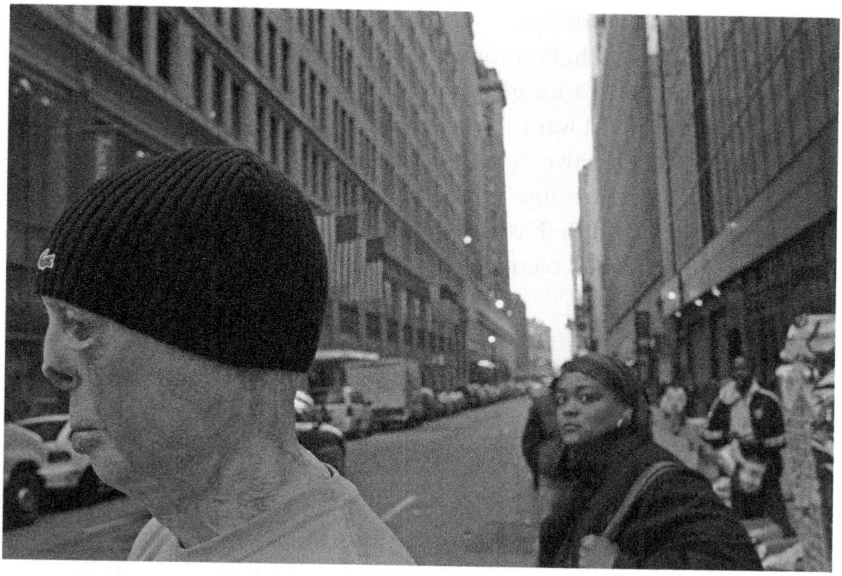

Fig. 12. Stuart Griffiths, British soldier (who was seriously injured in Afghanistan) on a charity walk, New York, 2008. (© Stuart Griffiths Photographs.)

tained third-degree burns over 70 percent of his body after the armored vehicle he was driving was ambushed by the Taliban in Helmand Province in 2006. His fiancée, Michelle, kept vigil at his bedside for three months as he lay in a coma. It was another month before he was allowed to see his face: "There were just the two of us when I held the mirror up for him," recalled Michelle in an interview. "He told me he'd understand if I didn't marry him looking like this, that we could call the wedding off. But I didn't want to hear about him giving up. . . . If you look beyond the scars . . . like I do, Martyn is still there."[84]

Compton credits Michelle with his survival: during his long recovery she brushed his teeth, washed his face, and fed him like an infant. The couple finally married in July 2008: an event celebrated by the *Daily Mail* as "the most beautiful wedding of the year as scarred soldier marries his sweetheart."[85] In November the same year Griffiths accompanied them to New York City for a charity walk. One photograph (figure 12) shows Martyn crossing a street adorned with American flags. We see him in profile at the edge of the photograph, the disfiguring effect of his injuries plainly visible. Behind and to his right, a woman casts a sideways glance at the camera, and by extension at us. Aligned with the image's vanishing point, her distrustful gaze interrupts our own. When I asked Stuart what Martyn and Michelle thought of the photographs, he said he had "edited" the prints before giving them a set: selecting "happy" images, the things they would want to remember.[86] Seeing the series as a whole complicates this selective remembering, and the tabloid image of the soldier whose "catastrophic injuries came to represent the tragic cost" of the war in the Middle East and whose "heroism in overcoming them" made him a "symbol of courage" for us all.[87]

A Meeting of Subjectivities

Linda Nochlin has remarked that what we look for in a portrait (unlike a medical image, mug shot, or press photograph) is "the meeting of two subjectivities": the subjectivity of the person portrayed, and that of the artist.[88] In this respect Berman and Griffiths have very different starting points. It is the autobiographical dimension of Griffiths's project that gives it narrative coherence and authority. This is especially evident in the long interview sequences in *Isolation* where we see Griffiths at work. "I think my own soldiering background has helped them open up to me," he explains. "They know I have respect and empathy for them and that is how I wanted to convey their injuries. I don't want to be brutal or sensational, but I do want to challenge the viewer with the reality of what serving your country means."[89]

Identification is not what Berman's photographs are about, and critics of *Purple Hearts* and *Marine Wedding* have seen her work as morally problematic on that basis. "Is there staging, not to mention exploitation, in 'stripping' the soldiers of signs of pride?" wonders Marcia Vetrocq in *Art in America*.[90] "Did they fight in a different war" than Greenfield-Sanders's veterans, "or does a documentary that honors survival require the selection of more resilient subjects?"[91] Likening the images of Ziegel to the late nineteenth and early twentieth-century portrayals of sideshow "freaks," disability rights activist Samantha Wehbi regards *Marine Wedding* as both voyeuristic and eroticizing. "Representations of people with disabilities," she concludes, have become "'collateral damage' in Berman's bid to awaken American society to the brutalities of war."[92]

That Berman may (or may not) have felt "enormous empathy" while taking the photographs seems to be beside the point.[93] She edits herself out of the printed and recorded interviews so there is no sense of a dialogue. "I have no words in the book," she says of *Purple Hearts*: "It's all their words."[94] Her portraits do not stage empathy or pity, and they do not prescribe an emotional response for us. There is little sense of physical or psychological connection with the people depicted in *Marine Wedding*, and little intimacy between them. Asked in interviews about the subjective content of her work—how she relates to the person in front of her—Berman emphasizes the importance of the initial interviews.[95] Although she records them—and has used edited transcripts and video compilations in publications and exhibitions—it is clear that the interviews, which can last up to three hours, are part of the process of making portraits and not just an icebreaker or additional output.[96] For Berman, it is during the conversations that the photographs begin to take imaginative shape. For her subjects, they serve a different purpose:

> I would interview them [for *Purple Hearts*], and that would kind of put them back in Iraq, in their head. And then I would ask them to sit or stand in a certain place, inside their house or room, or in the front yard. And because the camera I was using [an old manual Hasselblad] is a very slow camera, and it's loud, they'd never seen this camera before. It slowed everything down. And they were basically lost in a reverie.[97]

Like Griffiths, Berman's theme is isolation: a state of existence that is revealed here as both psychological and physical. Referring to the square format of her photographs for *Purple Hearts*, she comments: "I always imagined that these subjects lived in a kind of a box."[98] When we imagine a soldier being wounded in battle, there is the physical impact, the explosion or gunfire, the tearing of flesh and shattering of bone. But in this iconic image of battle, says Berman, the soldier is never alone: he (it is much harder to call up an image of a female battlefield casualty) is surrounded by his friends and comrades. He is "taken care of . . . there's a structure in place." Berman's aim, with *Purple Hearts*, was to show that the real violence, "the real damage[,] is not in that moment."[99] Her photographs do not, as Dora Apel observes, "call a national patriotic audience into place." Instead, "The benevolent, impartial, paternalistic state implicitly constructed by Greenfield-Sanders's 'alive day' portraits is here implicitly represented as both utterly disruptive to "normal" civilian life and severely indifferent to that disruption."[100]

For all their intellectual coolness and emotional distance, however, there is in Berman's images of veterans an extraordinary attention to the material texture of the lives she observes (figures 13 and 14). The

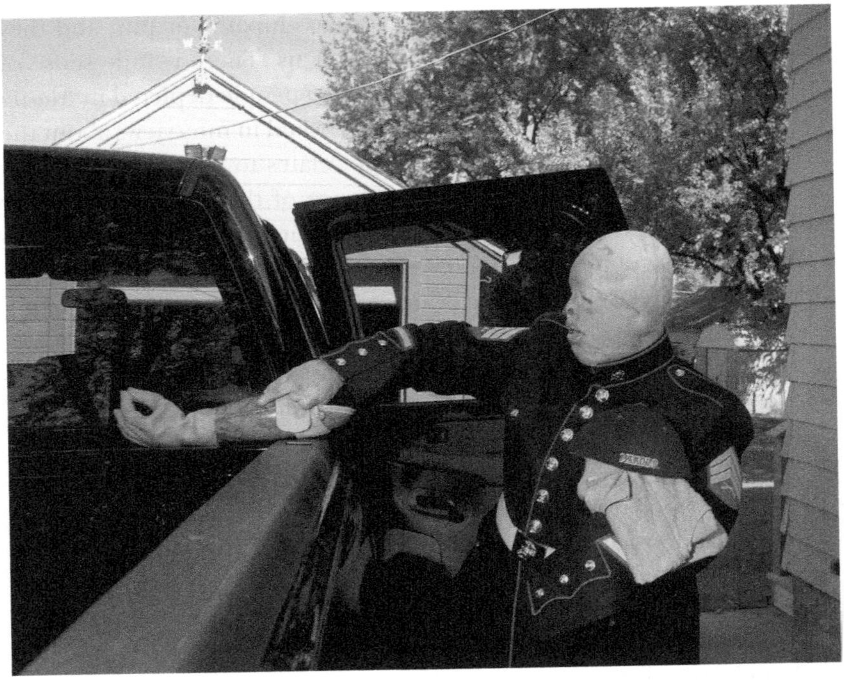

Fig. 13. Nina Berman, *Marine Wedding*, 2006. (© Photo by Nina Berman/NOOR.)

gleam of the buttons on Ty's dress uniform, the disconcertingly rubbery folds of his prosthetic hand, the stiff whiteness of Renee's gown and her carefully manicured fingernails: these details are replete with narrative significance. Ziegel's interior life may not be apparent in his face (which, captured in a photograph, can probably only signify trauma). Unlike Berman or his friends and family, we can't speak to him. The only identity we have access to is embedded in the material fabric of his life.

Berman's "subjectivity" may be less apparent than Griffiths's, but it can be discerned in the stylistic consistency of her photographs: in a certain formality of pose and composition, and in the deep, saturated colors that declare a distance from the documentary look. "I don't believe in the notion of the objective photographer," she has said.[101] Berman has received editorial commissions from *National Geographic*, German *Geo*, *Time*, *Newsweek*, *Harper's*, the *New York Times Magazine*, and other major news periodicals, but her technical and formal achievements are most apparent when the photographs are displayed, as large-format prints, in a gallery. I saw the wedding portrait in London at the Wellcome Collec-

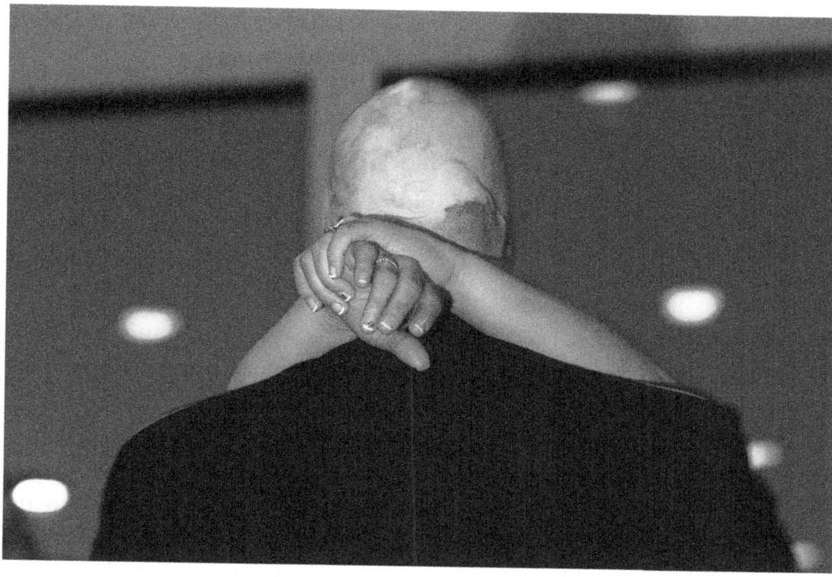

Fig. 14. Nina Berman, *Marine Wedding*, 2006. (© Photo by Nina Berman/ NOOR.)

tion's *War and Medicine* exhibition in 2008: it was the scale that immediately identified the photograph as "art" as opposed to photojournalism or studio photography. Formal beauty has come to seem suspect in the context of war, and Berman's inclusion in the 2010 Whitney Biennial drew some predictably disgruntled responses. One blogger described the Whitney show as "dehumanizing" because "it totally aestheticizes the work so that you think about [it] in terms of art and compositions rather than the human content."[102] But this criticism only holds if we can agree on what art is. What is "art" in the context of the Whitney or Wellcome Collection?[103] Part of the answer (especially in the last four decades) is that art is a means of interrogating beauty, representation, identity, and spectatorship.

In Griffiths's photographs of veterans, and in *Purple Hearts* and *Marine Wedding*, we can glimpse a different understanding of portraiture at work: one that invests narrative and emotional significance in nonfacial markers of personhood rather than relying exclusively on facial identity and expression. This is necessary, in part, because of the nature of the injuries depicted, but it also connects these images with an alternative history of portraiture in which presence and personhood are conveyed metonymically through the representation of corporeal details (hands, hair, skin) and material objects (relics, treasured possessions, the personal effects of the dead). These indexical strategies are very different from the visual logic of mimetic portraiture and personification. As Judith Butler remarks, the problem with personification (and, we might add, conventional portraiture) is that every time the human is "captured" in an image, "some loss of the human takes place."[104] For a representation to "convey the human," she suggests, it "must not only fail, but it must *show* its failure. There is something unrepresentable that we nevertheless seek to represent, and that paradox must be retained in the representation we give."[105]

For me, Griffiths's photographs go further than Berman's in admitting the impossibility of representing the face of war, and this perhaps explains his discomfort with "portraiture" as a label. There is, in *Closer*, no attempt to encapsulate the subjects in the usual ways (name, age, military rank, medical history) or to anchor the meaning of the images to specific memories or events. Nor is there any suggestion of having captured the defining image of the men and women he photographs: instead of the "true likeness," we find serial portraits that don't add up to a whole, but rather imply a fracturing of place and personhood. And the identities at stake here—including the photographers' and our own—are shaped by an almost infinite number of variables. Social class, gender, politics, military service: all of these factors frame the public response to these images as much as they inform the identities depicted. Berman's images, too, exploit our expectations of portrait photography while resisting the temptation to "consolidate the self portrayed." Unmoored from this traditional purpose, the portrait becomes a vehicle through which identity might be questioned, along with the concepts of likeness and ugliness.

When facial identity is masked or damaged, when the image of a face signifies trauma rather than character or emotion, then conventional expectations of likeness break down.[106] A good likeness is assumed to be different from an accurate depiction. It promises a distillation of the subjects' essence, a glimpse of their soul (or social status or moral worth). When the face is altered, however, it is usually perceived as a false image: not a good likeness. In place of the traditional notion of likeness—in these images—it is possible to discern a more dispersed and more contingent understanding of identity: as something that has to be assembled and managed, something that can be "spoiled," a fragile thing that can be made in a small-town photographic studio and unmade in a moment of unguarded staring.

CHAPTER 2

Aversion

A History

My leg? It's off at the knee.
Do I miss it? Well, some. You see
  I've had it since I was born;
  And, lately, a devilish corn.
(I rather chuckle with glee
  To think how I've fooled that corn.)

But I'll hobble around all right.
  It isn't that, it's my face.
Oh I know I'm a hideous sight,—
  Hardly a thing in place.
Sort of gargoyle, you'd say.
  Nurse won't give me a glass;
  But I see the folks as they pass
Shudder and turn away;
  Turn away in distress . . .
  Mirror enough, I guess.

—Robert W. Service, "Fleurette (The Wounded Canadian Speaks)"[1]

Disfigurement and mutilation were ubiquitous on the battlefields of World War I, in military hospitals, convalescent homes, towns and villages: an estimated 60,500 British soldiers suffered head or eye injuries, and 41,000 men had one or more limbs amputated.[2] At the specialist hospital for facial injuries near Sidcup in Kent, over 11,000 operations were performed on some 5,000 British and Dominion troops between 1917 and 1925.[3] Many soldiers were shot in the face simply because they had no experience of trench warfare: "They seemed to think they could pop their heads up over a trench and move quickly enough to dodge the hail of machine-gun bullets," wrote the American surgeon Fred Albee.[4] Military medical archives contain extensive visual evidence of these injuries. Until the past few years, however, these X-rays and surgical diagrams, photographs and stereographs, plaster casts and models were rarely on public display. It has even been claimed that they amount to a "hidden history" of World War I.[5]

During the war, visitors to the Queen's Hospital at Frognal, near Sidcup, would have been able to see Henry Tonks's drawings of patients before and after surgical reconstruction (figures 16, 43, and 49). Aside from these unusual studies, however, the disfigured face is almost entirely absent from British art. Francis Bacon's heads and portraits from the 1940s onward bear a strange resemblance to Tonks's studies of wounded soldiers, but there is a crucial difference: Bacon was painting his lovers, friends, and drinking companions; his violations of the human form are altogether more theatrical, more stylistically consistent in their violence. Neither the drawings by Tonks, nor the photographs in the men's case files, found their way into antiwar publications, as happened in Weimar Germany, and they never featured in the illustrated histories of the war.[6] As historical documents, they speak volumes about the kinds of injuries sustained in modern combat, and the medical response to these injuries, but it could not be said that they have been part of British cultural history in any broader sense; at least not until very recently.[7]

The focus of this chapter is the public discourse of bodily and facial reconstruction in World War I Britain. In the sources I will be concentrating on—newspaper and periodical articles, the reminiscences of doctors, nurses, and orderlies—a fairly consistent picture emerges. Facial injury provoked an anxiety that was acutely and specifically visual. Patients refused to see their families and fiancés; children reportedly fled at the sight of their fathers; nurses struggled to look their patients in the face.[8] Ward Muir, who worked as an orderly at the Third London General Hospital in Wandsworth, was surprised by his reaction to patients on the facial ward: "I never [before] felt any embarrassment . . . confronting a patient," he confesses, "however deplorable his state, however humiliating his dependence on my services, until I came in contact with certain wounds of the face."[9] A culture of aversion surrounded facially disfigured veterans of World War I. This collective looking-away took multiple forms: the absence of mirrors on facial wards, the physical and psychological isolation of patients with severe facial injuries, the eventual self-censorship made possible by the development of prosthetic masks, and an unofficial censorship of disfigured veterans in the British press and propaganda.

Most of the literature on disabled veterans has focused on limb loss and orthopedic care. Unlike amputees, however, these men were never officially celebrated as wounded heroes.[10] The wounded face, as Sander Gilman observes, is not equivalent to the wounded body: it presents the trauma of mechanized warfare as a loss of identity and humanity.[11] That radical facial transformation is likely to affect one's sense of self is self-evident. Less easy to tease out is the relationship between facial appearance and humanity. Why should disfigurement lessen one's *humanity* in the eyes of others? Gilman does not elaborate on this question, and Ward Muir and his contemporaries take the answer for granted. Facial casualties—especially those encountered by Muir in the weeks and months after they were injured—could not have responded expressively to those around them; their faces were not only visibly mutilated, but rendered inanimate. These attributes of the human face—the ability to convey subtleties of emotion or mood; to indicate or elicit understanding; to register another's presence—these are all compromised by severe facial trauma.

The neurophysiologist Jonathan Cole opens his book *About Face* with a moving description of one of his patients, Mary, an elderly woman who has lost all facial expression. The neurologists, nurses, and students discussing her case wonder if she is slightly demented. Although Mary's gestures betray her frustration—and she is still able to communicate in writing—it is difficult to gauge her comprehension because her face registers no emotion or understanding. Cole finds himself reflecting on Mary's case throughout the day:

> To be in the presence of someone without facial animation, and so almost without "face," had deprived me of a main discloser of others. . . . Without a face she as a person was all but invalidated. Her disease had opened up a seam between the face and self I had not realized was there.[12]

Faces do more than signify our individual selves: they are a common ground. In the words of the philosopher Maurice Merleau-Ponty (which serve as the epigraph to *About Face*): "I live in the facial expression of the other, as I feel him living in mine."[13] In the absence of the expressive face, words—written or spoken—might be called upon to fill the void. Nina Berman hints at this possibility when she says Tyler Ziegel would seem like an ordinary guy if only you closed your eyes. But language can just as easily be used to evade emotional contact, and in the final part of this chapter we will encounter some masterly performances of stoicism.

Despite (or perhaps because of) the common perception that facial injury entailed a loss of humanity, one sometimes finds the stigma of disfigurement tempered, in literature and journalism, by an idealized feminine gaze and touch. A woman's touch—that of a nurse, wife, or even a stranger—could transcend the dehumanizing and emasculating effects of mutilation. At the end of Robert Service's poem with which this chapter opens, the wounded protagonist is kissed by a girl who is visiting her injured brother, a French soldier. "Sixteen, all laughter and love . . . Half woman, half child,—Fleurette." Curious about the *malheureux* in the opposite bed, she discovers that he saved his men by smothering a bomb that fell into the trench. After kissing her brother goodbye, she goes to the other man's bedside. "*May I kiss you, sergeant?*" she asks.

> Then she kissed my burning lips
> With her mouth like a scented flower . . .
> God bless her, that little Fleurette!

"Could any woman come near that gargoyle without repugnance?" Muir wonders of one of the patients at the Third London General,[14] yet the saintly wife or devoted fiancée, the beautiful stranger and the attentive (and invariably pretty) nurse were enduring stereotypes in the wartime press. In a popular variation on this theme, a story in the *Sunday Chronicle* (previously published in the *Daily Mail*) recounts a wife's first visit to her wounded husband. He has not had the courage to reveal the extent of his injuries, and when she arrives at the hospital, the head nurse takes her aside to prepare her for the worst:

> "He told you of his wound?"
>
> "He said he was hit by shrapnel, ma'am, but not bad."
>
> Matron motioned her to sit down, and then, with an infinite pity in her face . . . told the little woman before her in a few words what Sergeant Bates in his agony of mind could not write.

> "So you see, Mrs. Bates," she ended gently, "you must be brave when you see him, because—he dreads this meeting—for your sake."

The visitor is ushered to her husband's bed, around which the Sister has hastily drawn a screen:

> She took one searching glance as involuntarily he turned his "good" side to her and then, deliberately choosing the other, she went right up to the bed, and with a hand on each shoulder kissed him—ever so lightly—on the worst scar of all.[15]

Disfigurement turns conjugal love into a parable of patriotic devotion, in which the wounds of war are salved—and the horror of war erased—by the reinstatement of domestic bonds. The *Sunday Chronicle* anecdote exploits the familiar image of the nurturing, self-sacrificing wife (or mother, or nurse) whose empathic gaze and touch overcome the memory and the physical trauma of combat. Like the accounts of surgical miracles, however, the fantasy of redemptive love has no parallel in the visual culture of World War I; not when the subject is facial mutilation. It is as though these narratives of sacrifice and hope might be cast into doubt by illustrations. Even Tonks was uneasy about the public interest in his medical portraits.[16] One might see reparative intent in his drawings, but as portraits they remain disquieting.

The argument advanced here rests primarily on textual evidence: what was said and written about disfigurement by nurses, orderlies, doctors, journalists, and artists. Although almost none of these sources were illustrated, they reveal a great deal about the visual culture of the injured body, if "visual culture" is taken to mean ways of seeing and imagining (and cultural prohibitions against looking) as well as visual artifacts. We begin, then, with the reasons and documentary evidence for a culture of aversion surrounding facial injury: the popular and professional perception of unsustainable loss. There are, I suggest, two cultural factors that contributed to the particular horror of facial injury during the Great War. One is that images of sacrifice (both martial and religious) had always relied upon the face as a signifier of valor or purity. Disfigurement, in other words, could not be accommodated within the available iconography of sacrifice. The other explanation is an abiding fear of syphilis: at the time still an incurable disease and associated, in its advanced stage, with facial lesions and deformity.[17] The new "face of war" closely resembled the old face of disease. Having historicized the anxiety surrounding disfigurement, we will turn to the discourse of facial injury during the Great War, beginning with several firsthand accounts by British soldiers who received treatment for facial wounds. The final section of the chapter contrasts the perceived indignity of facial mutilation with the sentimentalized and often idealized depiction of amputees, whose prosthetic limbs and altered bodies were highly visible in the wartime press. Facial casualties presented a medical challenge, to be sure, but the public spectacle of the mutilated face also provoked a crisis of representation; a "symbolic collapse," to use Julia Kristeva's term: a crisis that threatened to undermine the very concept of human nature in the context of social and economic upheaval and mass slaughter.[18]

Iconographies of Horror and Redemption

In one of the few publications to consider facial injury from the patient's perspective, Andrew Bamji remarks that the "horror of facial disfigurement is universal and enduring."[19] As the consultant archivist at Queen Mary's Hospital and curator of the Gillies Archives, Bamji was more familiar than most with the visual evidence of facial injury and its treatment in wartime Britain. The images in some twenty-five hundred case files—documenting the work of the British and New Zealand surgical teams at the hospital—are, he admits, "both disturbing and fascinating: suddenly one is transported from the calm realms of death to the indignity of disfigurement."[20] As a cultural historian rather than a clinician (Bamji was, until his retirement, an eminent rheumatologist), I instinctively raised an eyebrow when I read this. Why do we assume that the horror of disfigurement is universal? What has disfigurement to do with dignity? And why does the mythology of the "calm" (and dignified) death persist, despite what we now know of the ugly reality of war?

In early twentieth-century Britain, depictions of the wounded male body conformed to a Christianized iconography of heroic sacrifice that denied the "obscenity" of mutilation and death on the battlefield.[21] Photographs of the dead and wounded did find their way into circulation—despite the best efforts of the censors—but it was mass-produced prints like *The Great Sacrifice* (figure 15) that most people would have been familiar with.[22] Sold for a shilling with the Christmas 1914 issue of *The*

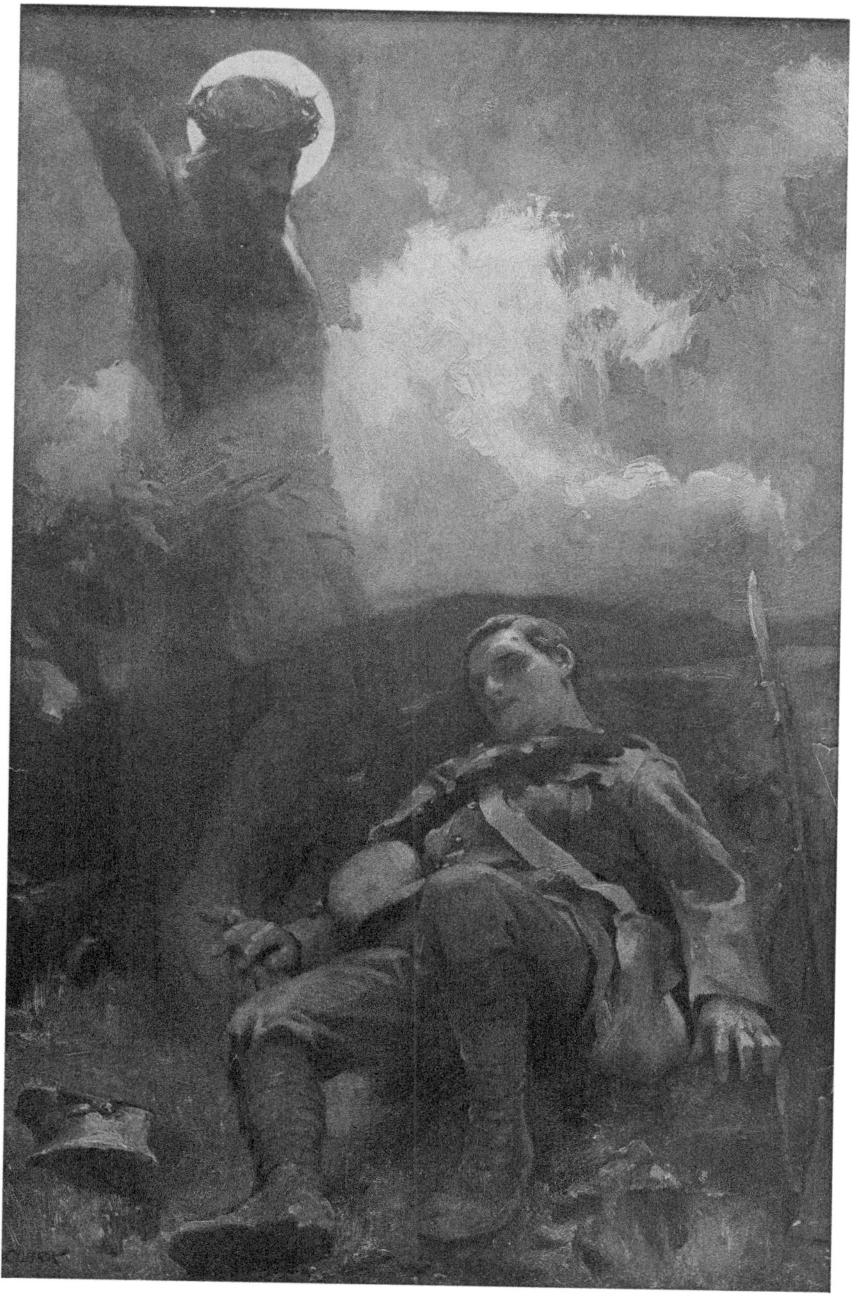

Fig. 15. *The Great Sacrifice* by James Clark, originally published in the 1914 Christmas number of *The Graphic.* Wellcome Library, London.

Graphic, the picture, recalled the chaplain Geoffrey Gordon, was at one time "to be seen in every shop window." For him, the image triggered less peaceful (and less dignified) scenes of carnage:

> A Young lad lies on the ground. A tiny bullet hole shows in his temple, and from it flows the faintest streak of blood. Over him hangs the shadowy figure of the Crucified. . . . Like the young lad in the picture, the man whom I saw die had a bullet wound in the temple, but there the likeness ceased. Here was no calm death, but a ghastly mess of blood and brains and mud, on his face and in the surrounding trench; and in the stark horror of the moment I could not see the Crucified at all.[23]

Christ's sacrifice was the exemplar: the ultimate model for death in combat.[24] "In war, the mere fact of dying was ennobling," notes Joanna Bourke, but one also had to look good.[25] In the posthumously published words of Arthur West, the awful truth was that the corpses were so "limp and mean-looking: this [was] the devil of it, that a man [was] not only killed, but made to look so vile and filthy in death, so futile and meaningless."[26] West and Gordon were concerned with the aesthetics of death as much as the fact of dying. Looking at the images reproduced here, one can almost itemize the attributes of a dignified death. The body should be whole: no missing limbs or gaping wounds are permitted; and while the head can be bandaged, the face itself must be undamaged and serene. *A Young Soldier Lies Dying* (ca. 1915) is a variation on the theme of the pietà (figure 16). In Dudley Tennant's version, on which this color halftone print is based, the young Madonna cradles the soldier's head in her lap as she gazes beatifically at his upturned face.[27] The last rays of a setting sun blaze behind her in the shape of a cross.

In Christian iconography the face is a site of transcendence, even (or especially) when the body bears the marks of suffering. The faces of the martyrs look beyond the corporeal world, beyond pain and death, to eternity. Immortalized by the likes of Pintoricchio, Carlo Crivelli, Lucas Cranach the Elder, Cosimo Tura, and other early Renaissance painters, the saints—each with his or her own instrument of torture—demonstrated that the face (and therefore the soul) could remain serene while teeth were pulled out, eyes were plucked, or the body was burned, beaten, or shot at with arrows. Beaded with blood and contorted in pain, the face of the crucified Christ is allowed to register suffering (theologically, it is imperative that he dies a "real death"). But

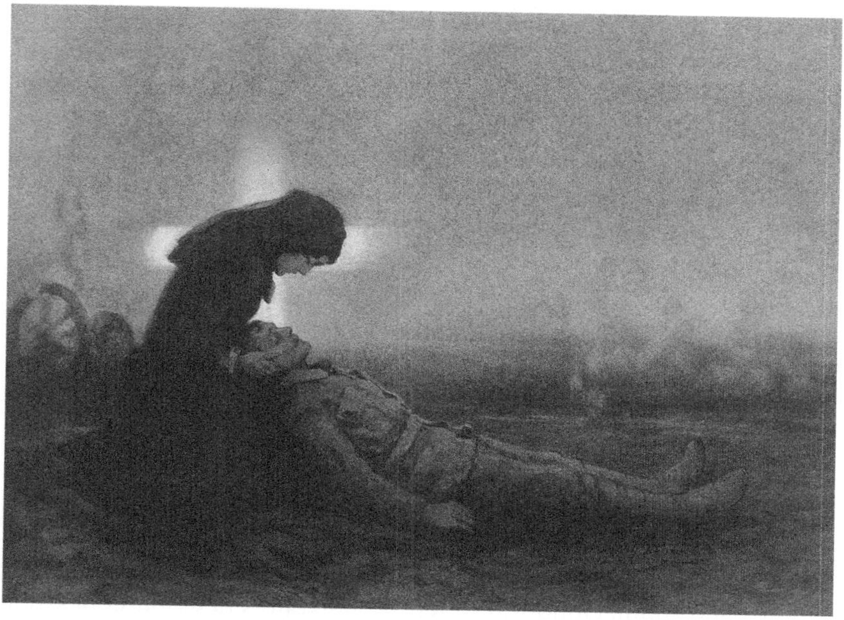

Fig. 16. Dudley Tennant, *A Young Soldier Lies Dying*, ca. 1915. Color halftone print, 32.7 × 45.3 cm. Wellcome Library, London.

Christ's face must still be beautiful, and the exceptions to this rule are truly shocking. Hans Holbein's cadaverous *The Body of the Dead Christ in the Tomb* (1521), in the Kunstmuseum, Basle, is one such exception. It has been the subject of lengthy exegesis: not least of all by Julia Kristeva, for whom Holbein's Christ is a harbinger of modern nihilism.[28] The most famous description, however, is in Dostoyevsky's novel *The Idiot*, to which Kristeva returns:

> The picture depicted Christ, who has just been taken from the cross. I believe that painters are usually in the habit of portraying Christ, whether on the cross or taken down from it, as still retaining a shade of extraordinary beauty on his face, a beauty they strive to preserve even in his moments of greatest agony. . . . In the picture the face is terribly smashed with blows, tumefied, covered with terrible, swollen and bloodstained bruises, the eyes open and squinting; the large, open whites of the eyes have a sort of dead and glassy glint. . . . How could [Christ's disciples] possibly have believed, confronted with such a sight, that this martyr would rise again?[29]

Just as the suicidal Ippolit, in Dostoyevsky's novel, struggled to reconcile Christ's visibly disfigured face with the doctrine of resurrection and salvation, the war-damaged face was incompatible with the image of heroic self-sacrifice. Rather than being seen as evidence of bravery or virtue, facial injury was feared as a fate worse than death. Disfigurement was a loss—a sacrifice—that could never be commemorated in a culture that, as Gabriel Koureas has shown, institutionalized the "sanitised and aestheticised body of the 'picturesque soldier'" while banishing—at least in the public sphere—the private memories of pain and mutilation.[30]

In *Illness as Metaphor* (1978) Susan Sontag speculated on the lasting impact of this Christian iconography of sacrifice on modern attitudes toward illness and disease. "Our very notion of the person, of dignity, depends on the separation of the face from body, on the possibility that the face may be exempt, or exempt itself, from what is happening to the body," she argues.[31] Polio, for example, marked the body, but it did not ruin the face. Compared to diseases like syphilis and leprosy (which, untreated, cause extensive facial disfigurement), the reaction to polio was relatively rational and "unmetaphorical."[32] Karl Rosenkranz's description of syphilis bears out Sontag's observation. In his 1853 treatise on the aesthetics of ugliness, the German philosopher contrasts syphilis with tuberculosis, that most romanticized of nineteenth-century diseases. The "putrescent sores," "nauseating eruptions," and "devastating bone damage" of syphilis give rise to "the most horrendous deformities." Though equally deadly, tuberculosis "gives the organism a transcendent air that makes it seem ethereal. . . . What a truly luminous sight it is to see a young girl or a young man on their deathbed, victims of tuberculosis," he exclaims. Just as illness causes ugliness only when "it modifies form in an abnormal manner," so too death "does not necessarily always make the features of the face ugly; it can also leave behind it a beautiful, blissful expression."[33]

In his own encyclopedic volume on ugliness, Umberto Eco makes the important point that the words we associate with beauty convey a sense of "disinterested appreciation," whereas synonyms for ugly often betray "a reaction of disgust, if not violent repulsion, horror, or fear."[34] As the following terms (from Eco's book) attest, the moral taint of ugliness is inseparable from its phenomenological effects. To be ugly is to be "repellent, horrible, horrendous, disgusting, disagreeable, grotesque, abominable, repulsive, odious, indecent, foul, dirty, obscene, repugnant, frightening, abject, monstrous, horrid, horrifying, unpleasant, terrible, terrifying, frightful, nightmarish, revolting, sickening, foetid, fearsome, ignoble, ungainly, displeasing, tiresome, offensive, deformed and disfigured."[35] Ugliness is not just beauty's other or opposite; it is, to quote Rosenkranz, the "hell of beauty."[36]

The conflation of aesthetics and morality is one of the cornerstones of the classical tradition, underpinning ideas of beauty in Western philosophy as well as Christian theology. Disease and deformity have for centuries been regarded as the outward symptoms of sin and evil. Nineteenth-century observers often described the disfiguring effects of syphilis—especially the deformed or missing nose—as a sign of moral corruption. Johann Friedrich Dieffenbach, who is widely regarded as the founder of modern plastic surgery, observed in 1834: "A man without a nose [arouses] horror and loathing, and people are apt to regard the deformity as a just punishment for his sins."[37] When the English surgeon and pathologist Jonathan Hutchinson documented the symptoms of acquired and congenital syphilis some fifty years later, he used the term "stigmata" to refer to the visible signs of the disease.[38] Sander Gilman (from whom I have borrowed these quotations) devotes a whole chapter of his history of cosmetic surgery to the physiognomy of disease. Perhaps the most iconic example of this idea is the grotesque figure of Erik in Gaston Leroux's novel *The Phantom of the Opera,* which was first published in English in 1911 and immortalized by Lon Cheney in Rupert Julien's 1925 film adaptation. Erik bears the stigma (in both the medical and social senses) of congenital syphilis: he was born with a diseased physiognomy. Behind the mask his skin, "which is stretched across his bones like a drumhead, is not white, but a dirty yellow. His nose is so little worth talking about that you can't see it side-face; and *the absence* of that nose is a horrible thing *to look at.*"[39]

By the close of the nineteenth century, Gilman argues, plastic surgeons had redefined disfigurement as an "aesthetic error."[40] Morality was still very much part of the equation, though: not because ugliness was an indelible mark of moral degradation, but because it could be—and therefore should be—corrected. We shall return to the moral imperative of surgical and prosthetic "repair" in the next chapter. First, however, let us examine the evidence that facial disfigurement continued to provoke anxiety in the context of war.

War and the Rhetoric of Disfigurement

It is worth reiterating, before we go any further, that this book (like Gilman's) is concerned primarily with the idea and representation of disfigurement. The private experience of men who were facially injured in World War I is much more elusive. On the occasions that they did put pen to paper, Gillies's patients were apt to be stoical and good-humored. "It is too late now to adduce directly the psychological effect of facial injury," Bamji writes, not least because "The men's own accounts, against all the odds, are remarkably cheerful."[41] The wounded were expected to exhibit fortitude, of course, to make light of their pain, and at the end, to die quietly.[42] "I've got a motto," went the popular music-hall song by Alfred Lester: "always merry and bright!"[43] We think of injury and convalescence as passive states—to be a *patient* is "to receive medical treatment"—but what comes across in the letters, diaries, and memoirs of the war wounded is the performative effort involved.

During their long periods of convalescence, the patients at the Queen's Hospital were encouraged to attend workshops and classes to improve their employment prospects and help them prepare for civilian life. Some of these activities—toy making and poultry farming, for example—are featured in newspaper and magazine articles; other skills included watch and clock repairing, coachbuilding, cinema operating, dentistry, and hairdressing.[44] Literacy classes were also offered, and it was in one of these, in 1922, that six of Gillies's patients wrote essays on the topic of "My Personal Experiences and Reminiscences of the Great War."[45] In these neatly penned exercises there is little evidence of despair: most of the men describe in detail the circumstances surrounding their injuries—the surprising "smack" of a bullet hitting the face[46]—and four of the six conclude on a positive note.[47] Aside from worries about pensions and employment, the consensus (among this small and self-selected group) was that it had been worth it. "I cannot say I am sorry I joined the army, as it has broadened my outlook on life," wrote Private Best. "So after all, I lost little, and gained much, through the Great War."[48]

In addition to these six essays, the Liddle archive at Leeds University contains several very detailed firsthand accounts by British soldiers treated for facial injuries. One set of papers comprises the typewritten recollections of J. G. H. Holtzapffel, along with a scrapbook containing a 1916 photograph from *The Tatler* of the young captain before his injury, and a press clipping from 1920 about wartime advances in plastic surgery. Indefatigably jaunty, Holtzapffel describes the sensation of being shot in the face as not "much worse than if I had a straight left from a middle-weight."[49] Upon feeling a little faint, he is put on a stretcher and carried to the aid post by four German prisoners, while a fifth prisoner provides shade with his helmet. A doctor's offer of morphine is declined and the patient is conveyed to the casualty clearing station, again offered morphine, loaded onto the ambulance train to Rouen, and from there transported to Le Havre and finally Southampton. On his way to London by hospital train he is surprised, reading his label, to find himself described as "Gun-shot wound. Face. Severe."[50] At the "Great Central Hotel" (as the Prince of Wales Hospital was known), Holtzapffel regards his damaged face in the mirror for the first time and can't help laughing, "for I had the finest pair of black eyes imaginable."[51]

The next few months are spent at the Sir John Ellerman Hospital in Regent's Park. A shipping magnate and financier, Ellerman had offered his large house, St John's Lodge, to the British Red Cross for use as a hospital for disabled officers. The hospital opened on January 27, 1917, with sixty beds, and closed in 1919.[52] Holtzapffel notes what a "marvellous place" it was, and that the VADs (Voluntary Aid Detachment members)—"all first rate girls"—provided the "greatest care and attention."[53] On one occasion, a medical officer prescribes champagne and oysters for postoperative complications.[54] Gillies finally makes an appearance as the consulting plastic surgeon, as does the sculptor Kathleen Scott, who oversaw the preparatory casting and modeling at the Ellerman Hospital. Intriguingly, her diary entry for November 4, 1918, reads: "At the hospital I worked on a man with a wonderful face and no nose. These men with no noses are very beautiful, like antique marbles."[55]

Patients were encouraged to "get up and about" as much as possible, and were permitted to leave the hospital grounds in civilian clothes (rather than the notoriously ill-fitting "convalescent blues" worn by those of lower rank).[56] A blue band on one arm ensured that the public would recognize the men as wounded officers, and on Armistice Day Holtzapffel and his friends were "simply mobbed by the excited crowd" on Regent Street.[57] When the hospital closed the following year, the remaining patients were transferred to the Frognal. With the war over and a new (if imperfect) nose, Holtzapffel returned to civilian life, resumed his career as an engineer, married, and started a family. He reminisces about summer holidays in the family bungalow on Selsey Bill in West Sussex, where, when the boys were young, they would dig pretend trenches in the garden and play "wonderful battles with their toy soldiers."[58]

A similarly buoyant outlook suffuses the letters written by Lance Sergeant Reginald Evans. From his daughter's brief biographical note, we learn that Reginald and his four siblings were brought up by their mother in Hemel Hempstead, and that before the war Reg was apprenticed to the Kent Brush factory. He had served in the Territorials since 1913, and received a Distinguished Conduct Medal for his part in a night reconnaissance mission on the western front. The first letter, dated February 16, 1916, is from Reginald's commanding officer to his mother, Mrs. Evans, informing her that her son has been wounded "rather badly" and praising his fearlessness and unflagging good spirits: "I have never met anyone so amazingly cheerful," Captain Whitfield exclaims, "the worse the weather and the more awful things were the more cheerful he would become."[59] This observation is borne out in the regular correspondence that follows. Despite being unable to eat or smoke, Evans tells his mother that she "needn't have the slightest worry" about him, but "will have to prepare [herself] to receive rather an uglier duckling than before."[60] "You wait till I come swanking home with my false teeth and artificial jaw," he writes a month after his injury. "I'll show some of you up."[61]

Still in hospital in France, Evans has his first operation at the end of March and admits to his mother that the procedure "has eased a lot of pain." His next letter to her, a week later, is full of concern for her health—"for the weather is so changeable and treacherous"—and emphatic in its reassurances that he is not in pain or danger. "Above all *don't worry*," he writes.[62] On April 13 he is finally back in England and waiting for a hospital train to the Cambridge Hospital at Aldershot (where Gillies's plastic surgery unit is based prior to the opening of the new facilities at Sidcup). "Everybody is extremely nice," he reports, "and I have been introduced as a hero . . . I can't help feeling glad in myself that not only have I *been* there but also that I have been wounded for my country."[63] Once at Aldershot, preparations for his major operation begin. Could she get some card photos of him printed, Evans asks his mother. He doesn't offer an explanation, but preinjury photographs were used by both surgeons and sculptors. On July 1 there is a surprise visit. The king and queen "just drove up [to the hospital] and said they wanted to see the 'plastics' wards. . . . Of course yours truly came in for a little attention." Letters sent in August and September, before Evans's return home, tell of escapades into town, a convalescents versus officers of the medical staff cricket match and a tea party at Nurse Oakes's in Farnham, where they "spent the afternoon drinking lemonade through straws and eating ices." Even a preacher's misguided comment during a visit to Waverley Abbey is conveyed with a playful sense of irony:

> Yesterday when Canon Cunningham was preaching he was saying that it was everybody's duty at a time like this . . . to cultivate these good looks and make themselves as beautiful as they could. It rather tickled

> me and I started smiling and to my horror saw that he had seen me. He continued "In God's sight those with scars honourably won were more beautiful than anybody and with them there were no aids to beauty needed" and so on and so on.

Bamji suggests that Gillies's patients "internalise[d] their memories."[64] Their suffering may not have been articulated, but it is our moral duty, he implies, to remember it. It is not my intention to excavate Private Best's stoicism or Evans's optimism, and we can't assume that Holtzapffel's joviality—practiced as it is—is evidence of denial or repression. Rather than attempt to reconstruct the emotional lives of these men, I want to interrogate the popular idea of facial disfigurement as "the worst loss of all"—a perception shared, then and now, by many in the medical establishment.[65]

Aside from medical case histories, the most detailed observation of facial injury and its treatment by an English-speaking author is in Ward Muir's *The Happy Hospital*, which was published in 1918. A corporal in the Royal Army Medical Corps (RAMC), Muir already had some success as a novelist and had written pieces for the *Spectator*, *Country Life*, and *The New Statesman*.[66] The final chapter of *The Happy Hospital* is devoted to the facial ward and its decidedly unhappy scene of human wreckage:

> Hideous is the only word for these smashed faces: the socket with some twisted, moist slit, with a lash or two adhering feebly, which is all that is traceable of the forfeited eye; the skewed mouth which sometimes—in spite of brilliant dentistry contrivances—results from the loss of a segment of jaw; and worse, far the worst, the incredibly brutalising effects which are the consequence of wounds in the nose, and which reach a climax of mournful grotesquerie when the nose is missing altogether.[67]

This passage is difficult to reconcile with Holtzapffel's and Evans's lighthearted self-portraits, or the farcical "Advertisements" page from the Queen's Hospital Thespian Society's souvenir program (figure 17).[68] *The Happy Hospital* would probably not find a publisher today: we have come to expect a more sensitive (and more euphemistic) treatment of disfigurement and disability. Indeed, one of the things that intrigues me about Muir's account is that the mutilated male body *was* written about, and imagined, in such graphic detail. It was showing (and looking at) the disfigured face that was taboo.

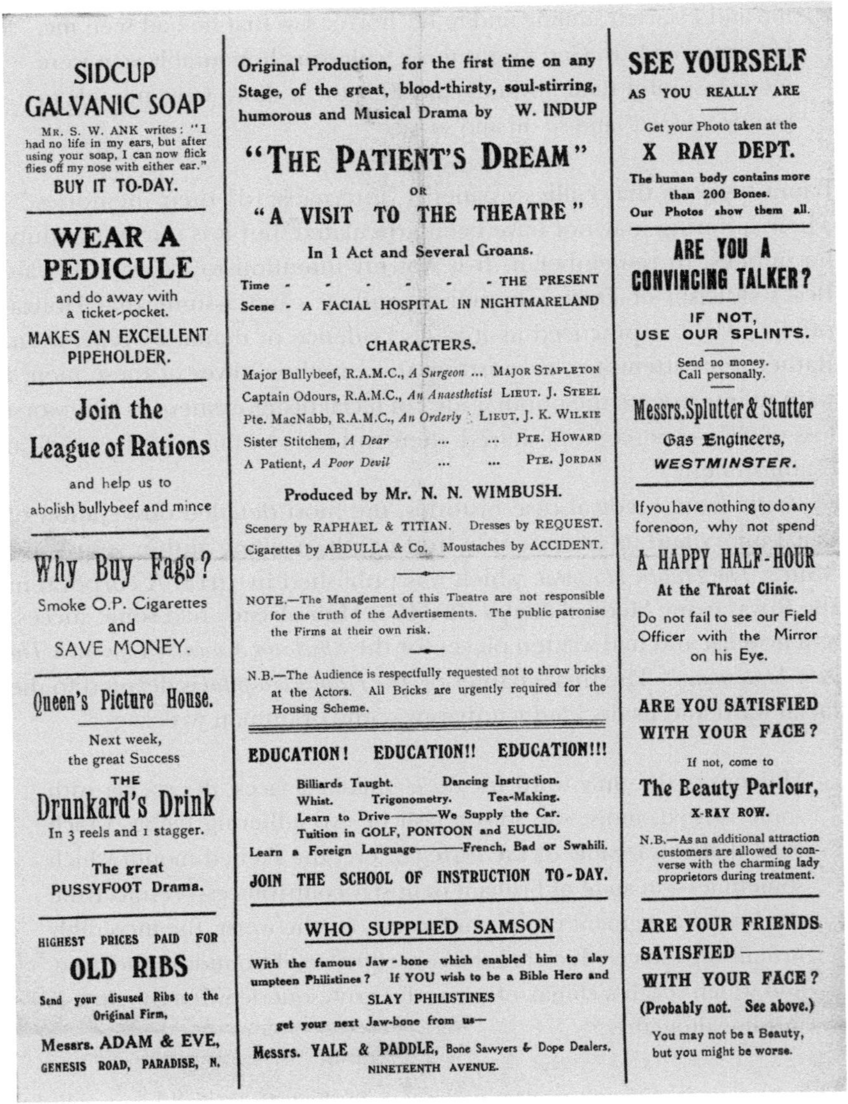

SIDCUP
GALVANIC SOAP

MR. S. W. ANK writes: "I had no life in my ears, but after using your soap, I can now flick flies off my nose with either ear."

BUY IT TO-DAY.

WEAR A PEDICULE

and do away with a ticket-pocket.

MAKES AN EXCELLENT PIPEHOLDER.

Join the League of Rations

and help us to abolish bullybeef and mince

Why Buy Fags?

Smoke O.P. Cigarettes and SAVE MONEY.

Queen's Picture House.

Next week, the great Success

THE

Drunkard's Drink

In 3 reels and 1 stagger.

The great PUSSYFOOT Drama.

HIGHEST PRICES PAID FOR

OLD RIBS

Send your disused Ribs to the Original Firm,

Messrs. ADAM & EVE,
GENESIS ROAD, PARADISE, N.

Original Production, for the first time on any Stage, of the great, blood-thirsty, soul-stirring, humorous and Musical Drama by W. INDUP

"THE PATIENT'S DREAM"

OR

"A VISIT TO THE THEATRE"

In 1 Act and Several Groans.

Time - - - - - - - THE PRESENT
Scene - A FACIAL HOSPITAL IN NIGHTMARELAND

CHARACTERS.

Major Bullybeef, R.A.M.C., *A Surgeon* ... MAJOR STAPLETON
Captain Odours, R.A.M.C., *An Anaesthetist* LIEUT. J. STEEL
Pte. MacNabb, R.A.M.C., *An Orderly* LIEUT. J. K. WILKIE
Sister Stitchem, *A Dear* ... ... PTE. HOWARD
A Patient, *A Poor Devil* ... ... PTE. JORDAN

Produced by Mr. N. N. WIMBUSH.

Scenery by RAPHAEL & TITIAN. Dresses by REQUEST.
Cigarettes by ABDULLA & Co. Moustaches by ACCIDENT.

NOTE.—The Management of this Theatre are not responsible for the truth of the Advertisements. The public patronise the Firms at their own risk.

N.B.—The Audience is respectfully requested not to throw bricks at the Actors. All Bricks are urgently required for the Housing Scheme.

EDUCATION! EDUCATION!! EDUCATION!!!

Billiards Taught. Dancing Instruction.
Whist. Trigonometry. Tea-Making.
Learn to Drive——We Supply the Car.
Tuition in GOLF, PONTOON and EUCLID.
Learn a Foreign Language——French, Bad or Swahili.

JOIN THE SCHOOL OF INSTRUCTION TO-DAY.

WHO SUPPLIED SAMSON

With the famous Jaw-bone which enabled him to slay umpteen Philistines? If YOU wish to be a Bible Hero and SLAY PHILISTINES get your next Jaw-bone from us—

Messrs. YALE & PADDLE, Bone Sawyers & Dope Dealers,
NINETEENTH AVENUE.

SEE YOURSELF

AS YOU REALLY ARE

Get your Photo taken at the

X RAY DEPT.

The human body contains more than 200 Bones.
Our Photos show them all.

ARE YOU A CONVINCING TALKER?

IF NOT, USE OUR SPLINTS.

Send no money.
Call personally.

Messrs. Splutter & Stutter
Gas Engineers,
WESTMINSTER.

If you have nothing to do any forenoon, why not spend

A HAPPY HALF-HOUR

At the Throat Clinic.

Do not fail to see our Field Officer with the Mirror on his Eye.

ARE YOU SATISFIED WITH YOUR FACE?

If not, come to

The Beauty Parlour,
X-RAY ROW.

N.B.—As an additional attraction customers are allowed to converse with the charming lady proprietors during treatment.

ARE YOUR FRIENDS SATISFIED —— WITH YOUR FACE?

(Probably not. See above.)

You may not be a Beauty, but you might be worse.

Fig. 17. Souvenir Program, Queen's Hospital Thespian Society, Sidcup, Friday December 19, 1919. (Courtesy of the Gillies Archives.)

"Very severe facial disfigurement" was among the injuries for which a veteran was paid the full pension.[69] As Bourke points out, from 1917 the Ministry of Pensions' calculation was made not on the basis of a loss of function or earning capacity, but in relation to a normative concept of masculinity. "Each part of men's bodies was allocated a moral weighting," she argues, "based on the degree to which it incapacitated a man from 'being' a man, rather than 'acting' as one."[70] Disfigurement exemplifies this distinction between "being" and "acting." Although severe facial injury usually resulted in loss of function, the horror of disfigurement—and payment of the full pension—was entirely about a loss of appearance. Men of officer rank or above were paid a higher rate of pension, not relative to their actual or potential income, but because of "psychological variables" that supposedly set them apart from the rank and file.[71] This implied hierarchy of suffering points to the unequal distribution of physical capital within society. "Physical capital" (the term used by Bourdieu) is glossed by the sociologist Chris Shilling as "the ability of dominant groupings to define their bodies and lifestyle as superior, worthy of reward, and as metaphorically and literally, the embodiment of class."[72] The idea that one's *face* is an embodiment of class and a form of capital—a resource, in other words—is perfectly familiar in the context of aesthetic surgery (although it is usually the female face that is seen as the legitimate object of cosmetic or surgical investment). Gillies regarded his young male patients in much the same way. Facial deformities not only cause distress and anguish, he observed, "but materially lower the market value of the individual."[73]

Ward Muir's description of the blind and partially sighted patients at the Third London General Hospital suggests that loss of sight was less horrifying (certainly for Muir) than loss of appearance. "If you want to hear the merriest banter in a war hospital," he writes, "visit the blind men's wards."[74] Disfigurement compromised a man's sense of self and his social existence. It deprived him of the "visible proof" of his identity, according to the *Manchester Evening Chronicle*:

> The torturing knowledge of that loss, while it lasts, infects the man mentally. He knows that he can turn on to grieving relatives or to wondering, inquisitive strangers only a more or less repulsive mask where there was once a handsome or welcome face.[75]

One of the earliest accounts in the press of the work being done by Gillies and his staff at Aldershot—an article in the *Daily Mail* from September 1916—set the scene in terms that were to become standard tabloid fare: "Nowhere do the sheer horror and savagery of modern warfare appeal so vividly to the mind and senses as in a tour of these wards."[76] Doctors and nurses who came into contact with facial casualties were also profoundly affected. "In all my nursing experiences those months at Aldershot in the ward for facial wounds were, I think, the most harrowing," recalled Nurse Catherine Black: "Hardest of all was the task of trying to rekindle the desire to live in men condemned to lie week after week smothered in bandages, unable to talk, unable to taste, unable even to sleep, and all the while knowing themselves to be appallingly disfigured."[77] Fred Albee's response was similar. In *A Surgeon's Fight to Rebuild Men* he concludes:

> The psychological effect on a man who must go through life, an object of horror to himself as well as to others, is beyond description. . . . It is a fairly common experience for the maladjusted person to feel like a stranger to his world. It must be unmitigated hell to feel like a stranger to yourself.[78]

When the Queen's Hospital opened in August 1917, the new facility and its patients received considerable attention in the press.[79] The physical and psychological isolation of the men was a recurring theme, as were the wonders of modern surgery. Patients often spent two years or more in treatment, undergoing multiple operations, and often returning for further operations after being discharged. These men were "The Loneliest of all Tommies," "the most tragic of all war's victims . . . half strangers among their own people, and reluctant even to tread the long-wished-for paths of home."[80] The Frognal estate's extensive and secluded grounds, including a hundred-acre farm, provided an ideal setting for lengthy convalescence (figure 18).

The *Morning Post* is typical in its emphasis on the "privacy and beauty of the place," which made it perfectly suited "for the purpose to which it has been put," for the patients "are almost condemned to isolation unless surgery can repair the damage."[81] To be in an ordinary military hospital meant "braving the streets, and the pitying stares or shocked, averted looks of passers-by."[82] Newspapers covering the opening of the new hospital reported that "many of the patients are so conscious of their affliction that they refuse to return to their homes and friends." This phrase is repeated in a number of articles, usually with the optimis-

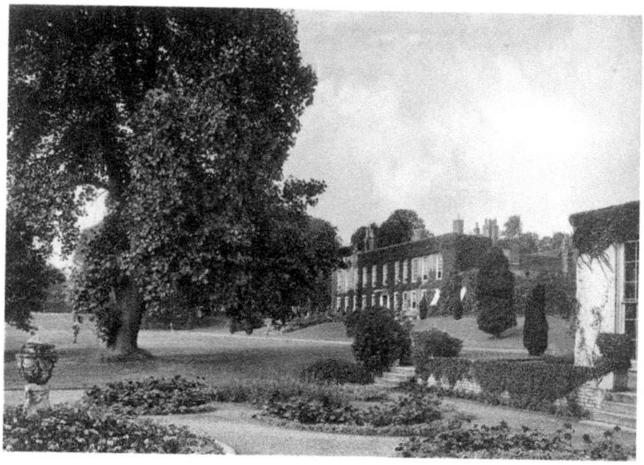

Fig. 18. View of the estate at Frognal, Queen Mary's Hospital album. Gillies Archives, Queen Mary's Hospital, Sidcup. (Photograph courtesy of the Gillies Archives.)

tic comment: "Happily the marvels of present-day surgery are such that cures can be effected in 90 per cent of the cases."[83]

At a narrative level, these brief and formulaic reports lead the reader from horror to relief. Scientific progress ameliorates the fear (perhaps more than the reality) of facial mutilation—and of course these articles were aimed at mothers, fathers, wives, and girlfriends of men who might well be sent home with their faces shattered "beyond description."[84] The morale of the troops was another consideration: on both sides of the war, severely disfigured men were judged unfit for service "for the reason that the psychological effect on other soldiers interfered with discipline."[85] The hospital page in the *Daily Graphic* predicts: "Soon the scientist will rival Nature herself in creating and rebuilding." By means of plastic surgery—"the most extraordinary medical discovery of this wonderful age"—"terrible facial injuries can be so patched up as to remove all horror and grotesqueness and make the sufferer quite normal again."[86] "If [Gillies] has not invented 'plastic surgery,'" enthuses another correspondent, "he has raised it to a magical level unknown before the war. He has enabled men to blush with cheeks covered with skin taken from their chests."[87] The *Kent Messenger* describes a surgeon arriving to perform his "Christ-like work" on the young hero whose face is so "grievously disfigured" that his own children flee from him in fright: the terrified children another stock anecdote in the rhetoric of disfigurement.[88]

Many such stories were published in illustrated papers, but the surgical miracles they describe are very rarely shown. Occasionally one sees bandaged men enjoying boyish pursuits of leapfrog or bowls, making woolly plush toys in the workshop, or tending the animals on the farm

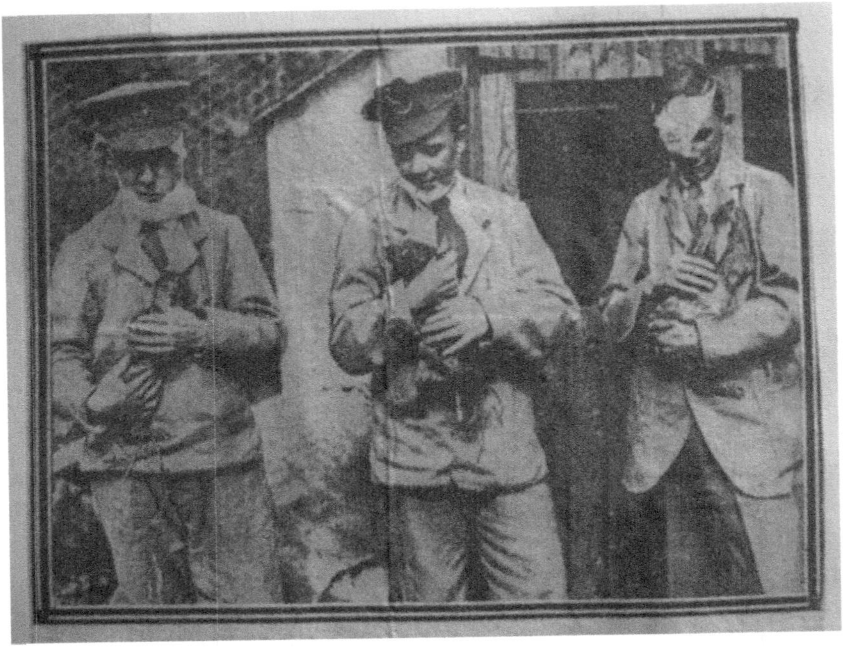

Fig. 19. June 12, 1918, *Daily Sketch*, 4–5. "Petting before potting—the men take much interest in the rabbits." (Reproduced with permission.)

(figure 19).[89] *The Toy-Makers' Shop* was also the subject (ca. 1918) of a painting by John Lobley (figure 20).[90] Hung in the Royal Army Medical Corps section of the Imperial War Museum's opening exhibition in June 1920, the painting's narrative focus is a diminutive monkey astride a pile of stuffing.

The quiet and contained domesticity of the scene contrasts sharply with the more conventionally masculine representation of amputees in the press and propaganda. As an official war artist for the RAMC, Lobley made tidy studies of the hospital's workshops (he also painted the commercial class and the carpenters' shop) that are unusual in their careful attention to individual faces, some of them visibly scarred. Here too, however, bandages suggest a process of healing and conceal the most disfiguring injuries. Muir was haunted in particular by the "healed" faces he saw—the men for whom no more could be done—and the "after" photographs in the patients' case files make for harrowing viewing. Not even Lobley's paintings hint at the psychological and physical trauma of facial injury. There was no clinical record of the patients' emotional condition, but anecdotal evidence suggests that depression was common. Accord-

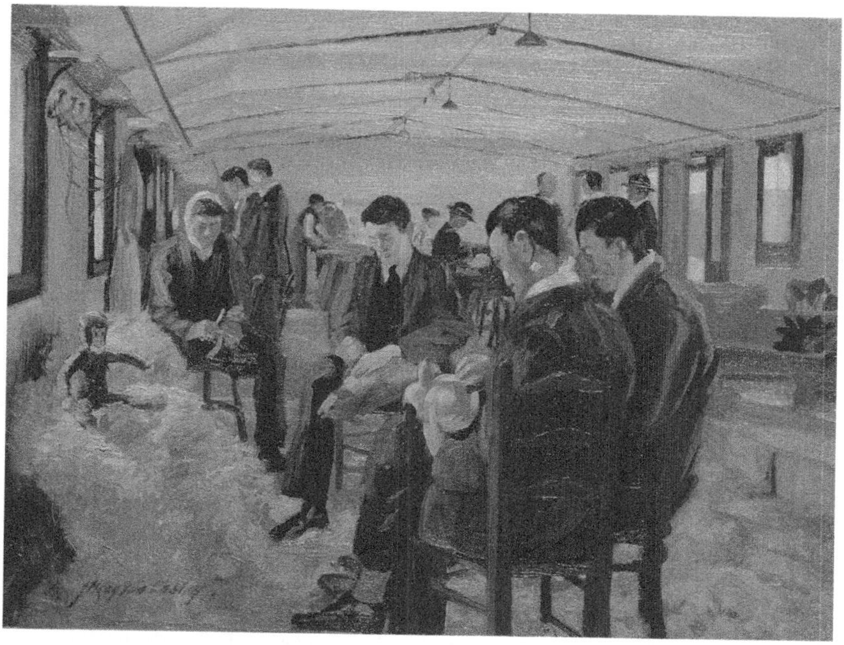

Fig. 20. John Hodgson Lobley, *The Queen's Hospital for Facial Injuries, Frognal, Sidcup: The Toy Makers' Shop*, 1918, oil on canvas, 45 × 60.7 cm. (Reproduced by permission of the Trustees of the Imperial War Museum, London.)

ing to Gillies, "Only the blind kept their spirits up through thick and thin."[91] Robert Tait McKenzie, an inspector of convalescent hospitals for the RAMC during the war, described the facial patients at the Third London General Hospital as "the most distressing cases" in military surgery:

> The jagged fragment of a bursting shell will shear off a nose, an ear, or a part of a jaw, leaving the victim a permanent object of repulsion to others, and a grievous burden to himself. It is not to be wondered at that such men become victims of despondency, of melancholia, leading, in some cases, even to suicide.[92]

Depression is also mentioned or alluded to in most of the news articles on the Queen's Hospital. The *Evening Standard* reports: "Not every one of the sailors and soldiers who have been severely wounded in the face or jaw at Frognal suffer from acute depression: but most of them do so."[93] In *The Times History of the War* (1916), facial injury appears in the section on shell shock and nervous injuries on the grounds that facial reconstruction, "while it belongs in a sense to the surgery of the war, possesses a psychological importance which is perhaps its chief consideration."[94] While the disfigured man "can live and can work," his life "is robbed of the greater part of its joy. He may be an object of pity, he is also, and he knows it, an object of fear. Men honour him, but they shun his company because his sorrow is too terrible to be viewed without pain."

The *Pall Mall Gazette* contrasts the mood at Frognal to that at the Queen Mary Auxiliary Hospital in Roehampton, where amputees were fitted with artificial limbs: "There is none of that depression [at Roehampton] which, however well diverted, attends in a more or less degree [*sic*] the fear of permanent facial disfigurement." Indeed, the *Daily Mail*'s medical correspondent declared Roehampton to be the "cheeriest place in England."[95] This is one of the most striking points of comparison between journalistic representations of amputees and those with severe facial injury: "disabled warriors" at Roehampton are shown strolling and running on their new legs, riding bicycles, playing cricket and football on crutches, chopping wood and playing golf with one arm.[96] They train to become carpenters, engineers, bookkeepers and chauffeurs; several photographs even feature amputees making prosthetic limbs in the workshops attached to the hospital.[97] Physical agility and manliness are reinscribed into the prosthetically remade body.

"More of a Man"

These accounts—implausible as some of them are—add texture to Bourke's assertion that the absent limbs of amputees "came to exert a special patriotic power" during the early years of the war, to the extent that the disabled soldier could be hailed as "not less but more of a man."[98] John Galsworthy, in his foreword to the 1922 *Handbook for the Limbless*, amplifies this sentiment: "The Briton has to be 'up against it,'" he wrote, "to be seen at his best—an expensive but thrilling characteristic."[99] An entire chapter is devoted to "recreations for those who have lost limbs," and includes bicycling, riding, boxing, and billiards for the one-armed. Those who were "sick" (physically or mentally) had to live with the suspicion of malingering; the "wounded," however, bore the visible proof of their valor and sacrifice.[100]

There is a paradox here: as Mary Guyatt points out, amputation was "one of the most visible reminders of war." Only by concealing the loss could the country "begin to move forward seemingly cleansed and guilt-free."[101] And yet, looking through the press clippings from Roehampton hospital, one is struck by the *lack* of concealment of absent and artificial limbs in comparison to facial disfigurement. Artificial legs in particular were presented as objects of superior craftsmanship as well as utility in much of the trade literature Guyatt considers; what is perhaps more surprising is the visual display of bodily reconstruction in the illustrated press. In two photographs published in the *Illustrated London News* in October 1915 (figures 21 and 22), we see the final adjustments being made to a full-length, polished, and ready-shod wooden leg.[102] The recipient looks on, his empty trouser leg folded loosely at the hip ready for the limb to be fitted. In the second image, another young man stands confidently—almost defiantly—without support, his trousers rolled above the knee to reveal a pair of brand new artificial legs.

The rhetorical and physical repair of limbless servicemen answered to a number of imperatives: military and economic as well as social and personal; but as the war continued, and its human toll became increasingly apparent, attitudes toward disabled soldiers inevitably began to change.[103] The economic cost of postwar reconstruction and competition for employment tipped the balance further against veterans who were dependent on the state for their limbs and livelihood. Writing in the inaugural issue of *Reveille* in 1918, Galsworthy predicted: "When the war is over, the cruel force of industrial competition will come into fuller play than ever before." "What sort of land will it be," he goes on to ask, if "five and ten years hence, tens of thousands of injured in this long tragedy are drifting unhappily among us, without anchorage of permanent, well-paid, self-respecting work?"[104]

The Victorian work ethic was central to the concept of rehabilitation, particularly the powerful association between working-class masculinity and skilled labor.[105] There was little expectation that single men disabled or disfigured in the war would find fulfillment in marriage (though of course many did), but for married men, financial independence was a precondition for their return to domestic masculinity.[106] An illustrated story in the *Graphic* celebrates the transformation of pitiful "creatures" into men. On the title page, under an ornate banner proclaiming "Roehampton: The House of Redemption," the society writer Margaret Chute conjures a cheerful scene, "full of life and merry voices," where "on every wall and notice board may be seen these words, 'Learn a Trade!'"

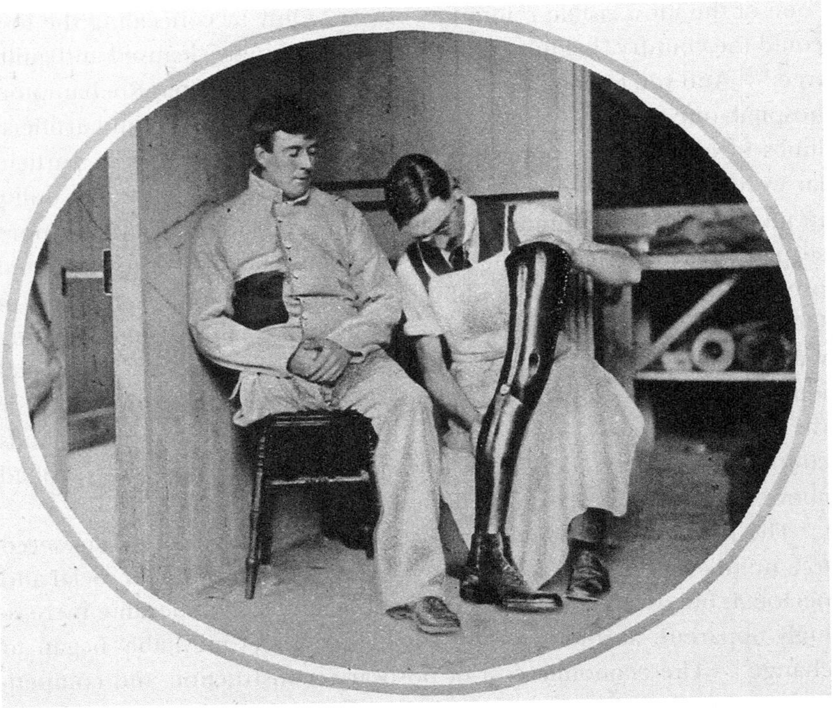

Fig. 21. *Illustrated London News,* October 16, 1915. "Artificial limbs for wounded British soldiers: adjusting a new leg at Roehampton House after a first trial-walk with it" (© Illustrated London News Ltd / Mary Evans.)

> They come to Roehampton in thousands, disabled, crippled men. They leave, redeemed by human skill; no longer useless, limbless creatures, but men anxious and fit to work again and take a place in the world of workers. That is the mission of this House of Redemption.[107]

That the wartime press functioned as an organ of propaganda is beyond dispute: one finds all kinds of distortion, from colorful embellishment to blatant untruth—often in the interests of charity. The *Evening Standard*'s recreation fund paid for gramophones, books and magazines, theatrical productions and concerts, picnics, cinema exhibitions, and games at Sidcup.[108] Harold Gillies applauded "the helpful way in which the great newspaper chiefs . . . banged the drum for our cause in the early days. It did a great deal of good."[109] If we want to know more about the actual experience of disability or disfigurement, we clearly have to look else-

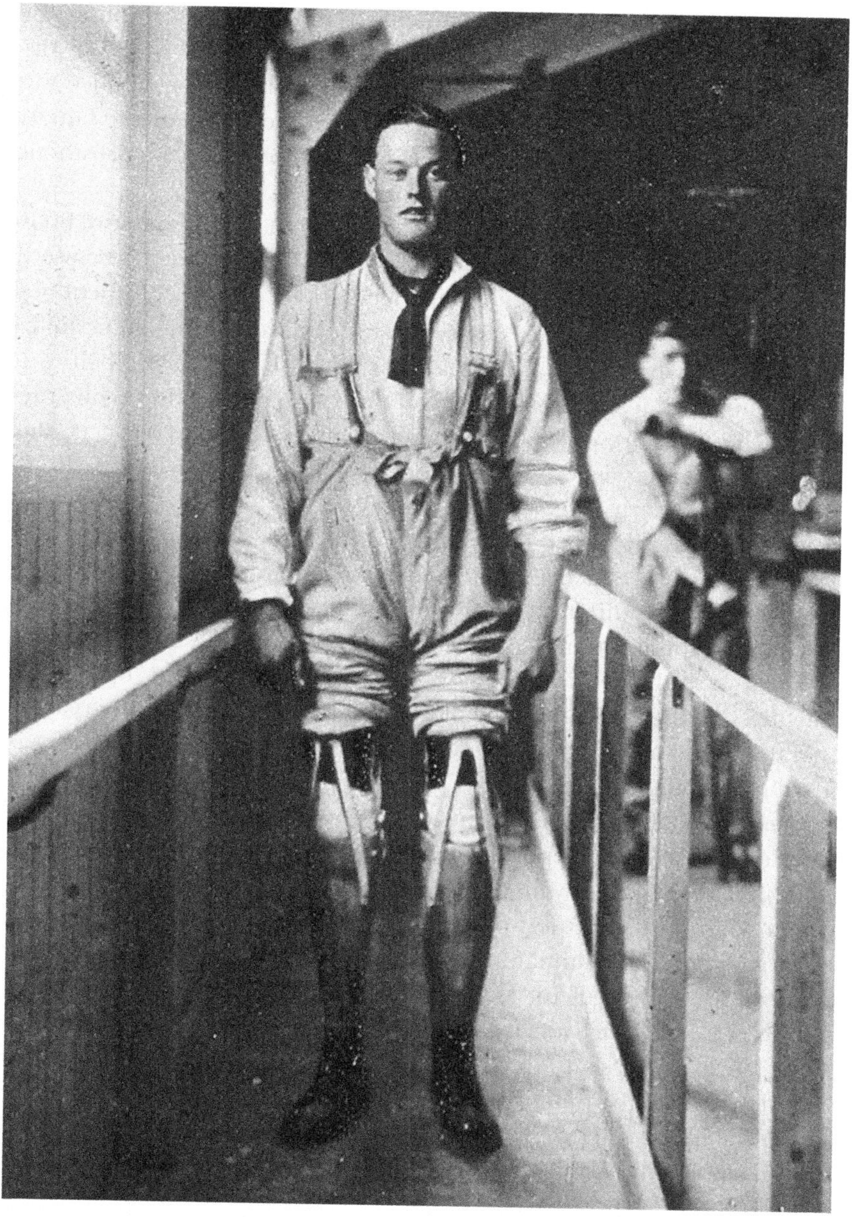

Fig. 22. *Illustrated London News,* October 16, 1915. "Making his first attempt to walk with the new limbs: A wounded soldier at Roehampton House with artificial legs." (© Illustrated London News Ltd / Mary Evans.)

where. But despite, or because of, their sensationalism and sentimentality, these sources reveal the ways in which the mutilated body was discursively remade, and the extent to which the burden of sacrifice was lessened by the idea of the marvels of modern medicine, or the fantasy of prosthetic repair. From this perspective, rhetoric itself has a prosthetic function: it is an "artificial substitute for lost parts."[110]

It has been suggested in this chapter that within this discourse of bodily sacrifice and repair, facial mutilation presents a problem because it concerns the identity of the embodied self, rather than bodily function—*being* a man, in other words, rather than *acting* as one. Prosthetic limbs were generally perceived as mechanical/functional objects (albeit with an aesthetic dimension), but the surgical and prosthetic reconstruction of the face presented different challenges. In many respects, this was a new frontier, where the modern war machine met human flesh, and where modern surgery met the uniquely dehumanizing effects of facial injury. Medicine could repair the mutilated body up to a point. It could return it to active service or to some kind of productive labor, but art offered a different kind of advantage: it could humanize. Gillies's famous description of modern plastic surgery as a "strange new art" points toward this sensibility. He was, writes his biographer, "uplifted by the idea that the activities of the plastic surgeon were essentially creative, that they demanded the vision and the insight of the artist."[111] One finds a similar fascination with the "art" of facial reconstruction in contemporary accounts of Francis Derwent Wood's portrait masks (the subject of chapter 3). The *Times* reported "magical results" being achieved "by the provision of masks . . . which will so far defy detection as to enable the owner to go out into the world again without shrinking." Thus might one "rob war of its ultimate horror."[112] In Wood's case, the encounter between art and medicine was largely accidental: confronted with the failure of reconstructive surgery, the "hopeless cases," he took up the challenge as only a sculptor could. For him, and for many of his contemporaries, art had the potential to overcome the loss of identity associated with facial injury, and to humanize those whose bodies bore the proof of war's essential inhumanity.

CHAPTER 3

Repairing War's Ravages

London

The Imperial War Museum houses some twenty-three hundred photographs by Horace Nicholls (1867–1941), most of them taken between July 1917 and November 1918.[1] Although Nicholls had made his name as a photojournalist during the Boer War, his request to cover the western front had been turned down. Instead, as "Official Photographer of Great Britain," he was commissioned by the propaganda bureau at Wellington House to make an official record of the war at home: the great munitions factories and shipyards, training camps, new recruits and soldiers on leave, the substitution of women in trades and services ranging from chemical engineering to grave digging. Although much of his work appeared in the wartime press and propaganda, most of these photographs remained unpublished. In the Imperial War Museum's Photograph Archive are twelve prints documenting the making of facial prostheses at the Third London General Hospital in Wandsworth.[2] These days they are easiest to find online, by typing "plastic surgery" into the IWM's search engine. Looking for the prints in the bound albums housed in the museum's All Saints Annexe in South London is more circuitous. Renumbered and undated, the group is likely to be discovered unexpectedly among more familiar scenes of munitionettes at their machines and portraits of women in uniform. Nicholls included descriptive captions under the heading "Repairing war's ravages: renovating facial injuries." Even without catalog numbers the narrative sequence would be clear. There are two sets of pictures, variations on the theme of reconstruction, each series centered on the prosthetic repair of a disfigured soldier.

The first four photographs (figures 23 to 26) show a shelled, ivy-covered building; a young man in a suit and tie with a deep triangular indentation between his eyes; the same man, now wearing spectacles and seemingly whole; and a thin crescent of time-fuse dated December 30, 1915, and measuring 2½ inches. A caption explains that the fragment, lodged behind the soldier's cheek, was massaged out through the entry wound without further damage to the face. Time-fuse and wound are visually linked to the ragged hole punched in the facade of the building. The juxtaposition of architectural and human facades has the effect of amplifying the force of the injury, but it also makes prosthetic "repair" a metonym for reconstruction as a whole: if flesh and bone can be so finely replicated, there surely is hope for crumbling masonry, splintered wood, and churned earth.

The second vignette (figures 27 to 31) unfolds in more detail, documenting the collaborative process of mask-making in the specialist studio set up by the sculptor Francis Derwent Wood (most famous now for his nine-foot bronze David atop the Machine Gun Corps Memorial at Hyde Park Corner).[3] Wood had joined the Royal Army Medical Corps as an orderly at the Third London General in 1915, along with several other members of the Chelsea Arts Club. He revolutionized the Plaster and Splints department and persuaded the hospital's commanding officer, Lieutenant Colonel H. Bruce Porter, to support his idea to make painted metal masks for severely disfigured servicemen.[4] The "Masks for Facial Disfigurements Department" was envisaged as a Roehampton for facial casualties, and by April 1916 Wood was recruiting patients from other military hospitals.[5] "My work begins where the work of the surgeon is completed," he reported in *The Lancet* the following year:

> When the surgeon has done all he can to restore functions . . . I endeavour by means of the skill I happen to possess as a sculptor to make a man's face as near as possible to what it looked like before he was wounded.[6]

There are cases, he adds, "which only the hand of the sculptor can deal with, or hands trained to serve both plastic and sculptural manipulations."[7] Wood's aim was to meticulously re-create the patient's original

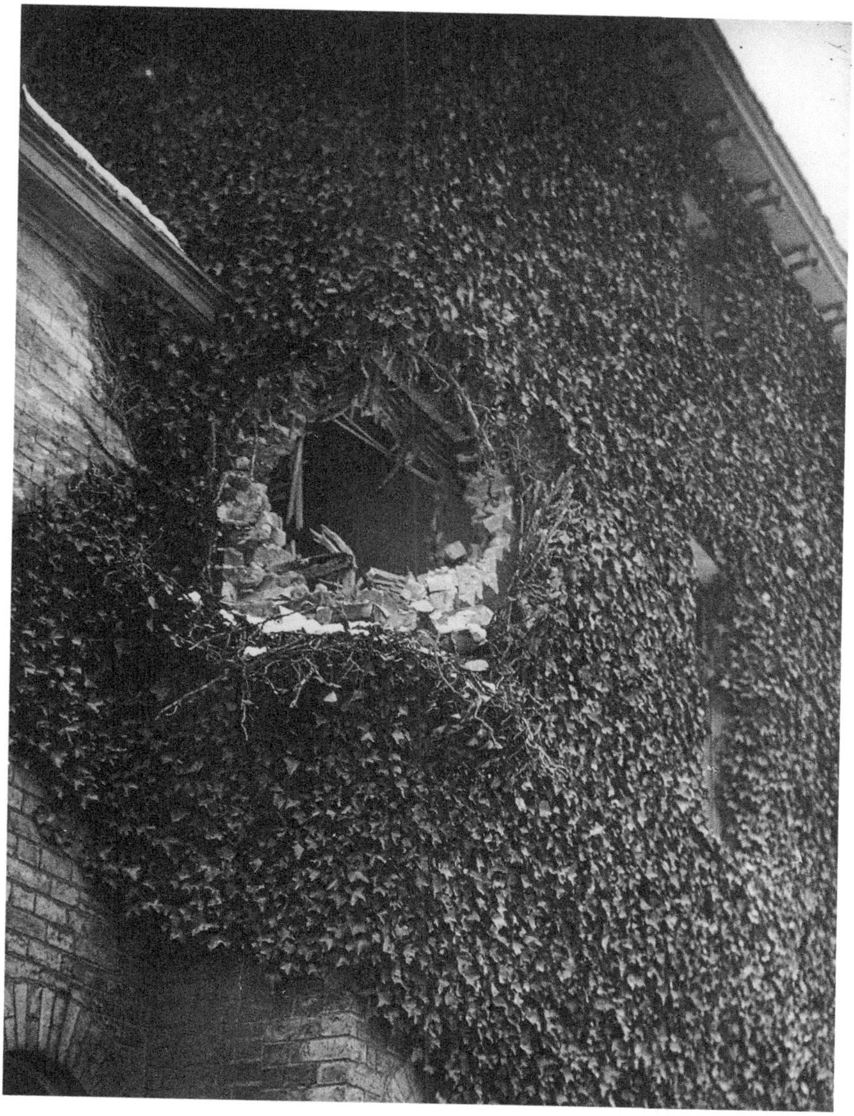

Fig. 23. Horace Nicholls, Germany's War on Open Towns. Imperial War Museum, Q.30.448. (Photograph courtesy of the Imperial War Museum, London.)

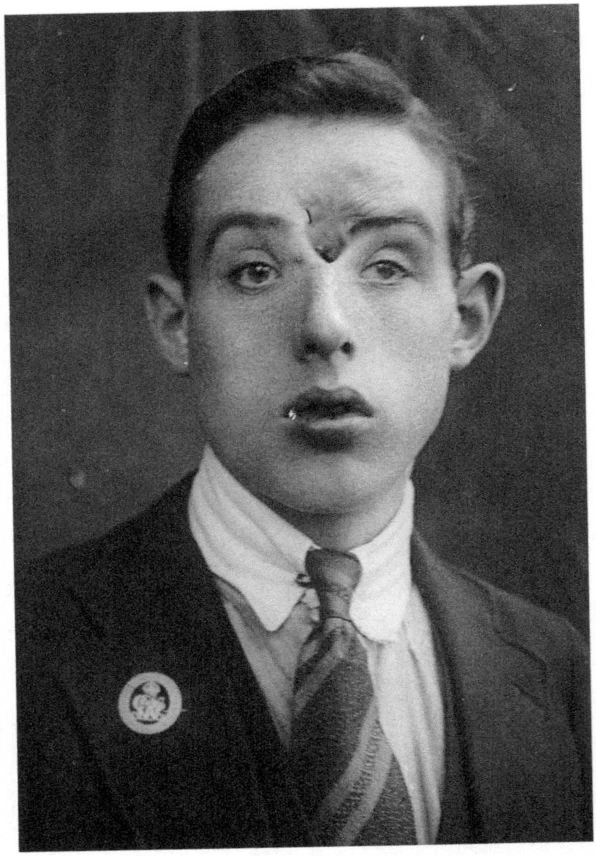

Fig. 24. Horace Nicholls, Repairing war's ravages: renovating facial injuries. A British soldier wounded between the eyes by a piece of time-fuse, which lodged at the back of his cheek. It was extracted by massage without injury to the cheek. Imperial War Museum, Q.30.449. (Photograph courtesy of the Imperial War Museum, London.)

appearance from his remaining features and preinjury photographs (often given as a keepsake to a wife or sweetheart). If an eye was missing, he tried to match the original color from the remaining eye or, failing that, from a relative's description, painting the reverse of a glass blank, or directly onto the plate.

The "Tin Noses Shop," as it became known, employed in addition to Wood three sculptors, a casting specialist, and a plaster-mold maker. In Nicholls's photographs we see plaster of Paris being applied to a patient's oiled face by two assistants, the initial mold drying in place and, once set, being checked for imperfections. Several steps are omitted: in the *Lancet* article, Wood describes how a clay or plasticine squeeze would be taken from this initial cast in order to produce a positive model of the face; a second cast and model would then be made as the absent

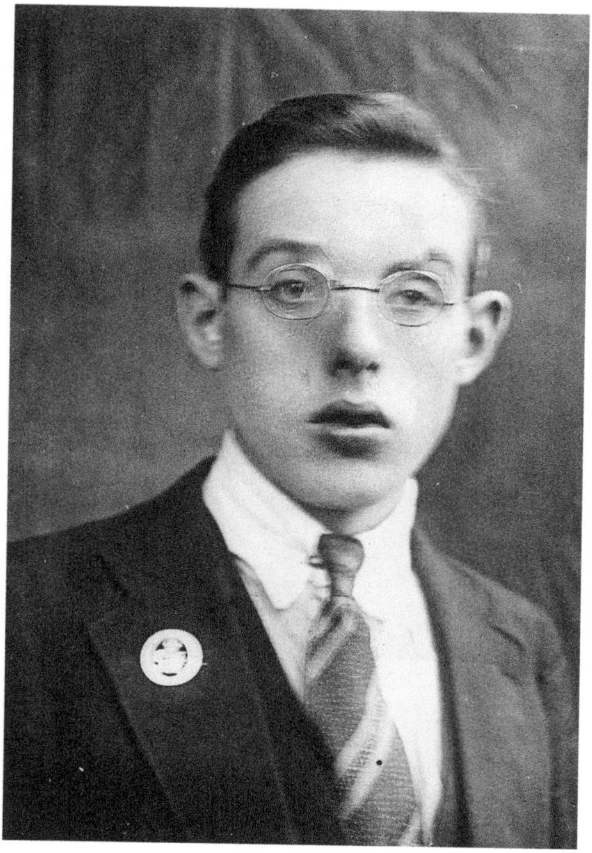

Fig. 25. Horace Nicholls, Repairing war's ravages: renovating facial injuries. The patient after a plate was fixed for the spectacles to cover the wound. The sculptor was Captain Derwent Wood, R.A., 3rd London General Hospital. Imperial War Museum, Q.30.450. (Photograph courtesy of the Imperial War Museum, London.)

features were carefully restored before final casting and adjustment, if necessary, to take an artificial eye. Nicholls's next photograph shows the patient regarding his ghostly plaster double, although the eyes at this stage are still closed. On this plaster mask a paper-thin copper electrotype shell would have been deposited, coated with silver, and painted to match the texture and tone of the patient's skin. Cream-colored bath enamel provided a good base for Caucasian skin, and the sheen of oily skin was replicated with varnish "rubbed down to match" the patient's complexion. Rather than use hair for eyebrows and lashes, Wood found that the results were better if he painted the eyebrows onto the plate, and used thin metallic foil for the eyelashes, which he would cut into fine strips, tint, curl, and solder in place.[8] In the final shots we see Wood with his palette and brush completing his artwork and examining the fin-

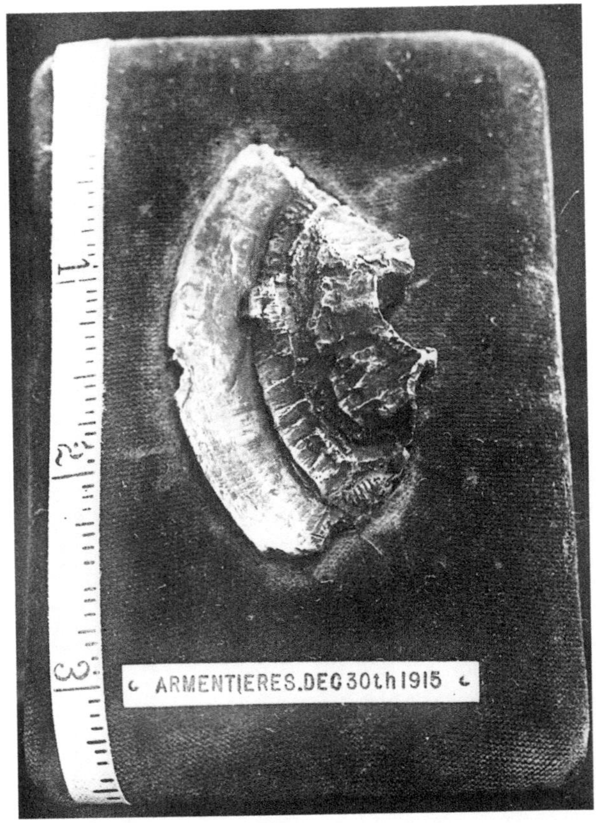

Fig. 26. Horace Nicholls, The piece of time-fuse which caused the wound. Imperial War Museum, Q.30.451. (Photograph courtesy of the Imperial War Museum, London.)

ished plate, a perfect section of cheek and eye. Two further photographs depict a row of casts and an array of new features in various stages of completion (figures 32 and 33).

Each plate took around a month to complete: mask-making was an individualized, highly skilled, and labor-intensive activity.[9] Unlike the manufacture of prosthetic limbs, there were no standardized parts, no economies of scale or mechanized production processes.[10] Considerable skill and expense was devoted to an object that did not, as Wood himself points out, restore function to the patient or alleviate his physical suffering.[11] What they could do, he suggests, is lessen a patient's psychological pain and social isolation:

> The patient acquires his old self-respect, self-assurance, self-reliance, and, discarding his induced despondency, takes once more to a pride in his personal appearance. His presence is no longer a source of melancholy to himself or of sadness to his relatives and friends.[12]

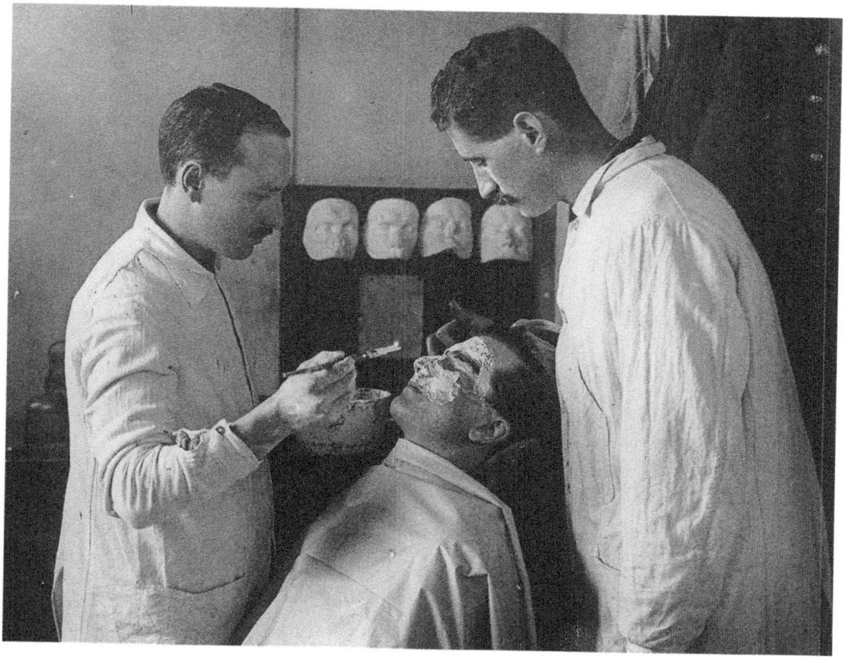

Fig. 27. Horace Nicholls, Applying the first coat of plaster for the purpose of taking the mould of patient's face, who has been blinded in one eye. The patch is to restore that side of the face which has been disfigured. Imperial War Museum, Q.30.452. (Photograph courtesy of the Imperial War Museum, London.)

This claim is repeated in *The Times History of the War*, which reported on Wood's innovations in facial casting and modeling in 1916. Marveling at the "dramatic quality" of the masks being produced for disfigured soldiers, the writer quotes at length from an earlier article by Wood, explaining the process of casting, modeling, and painting the plates, and remarking that by virtue of the sculptor's art, "that which was unbearable to the eyes became once again normal in appearance."[13] Returning to the subject of "facial restoration" in 1917, the happy coincidence of medicine and art is once again featured in *The Times History*. Unlike earlier attempts to make prosthetic masks, which "were usually obvious imitations and very unsightly," the new portrait masks were finely crafted by "an artist of repute." No longer were patients required to choose "from stock patterns": instead, each face was, as far as possible, "restored" to its former appearance.[14]

The Hunterian Museum at the Royal College of Surgeons in London has on display a rare example of a pre–World War I mask worn by a

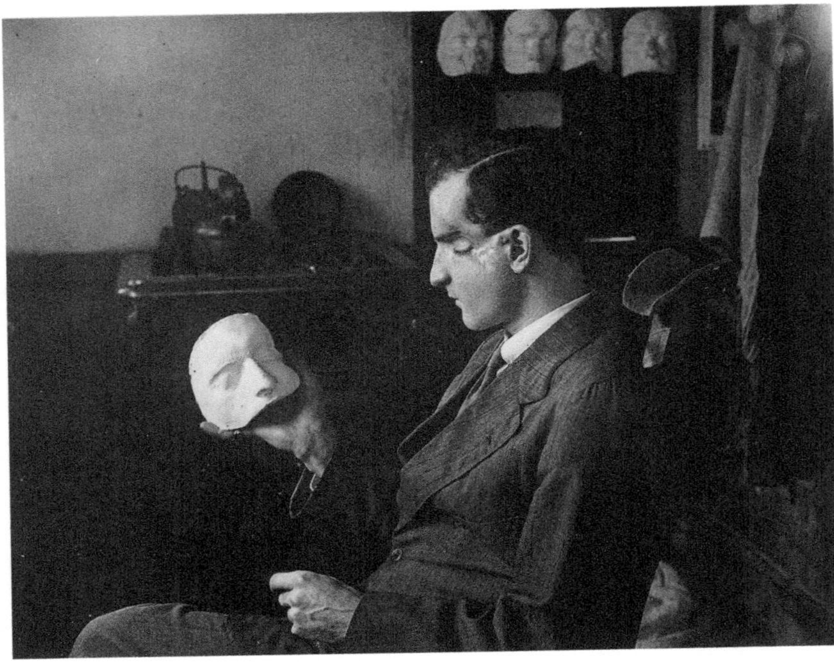

Fig. 28: Horace Nicholls, The patient examining the mould of his own face. Imperial War Museum, Q.30.455. (Photograph courtesy of the Imperial War Museum, London.)

civilian, William Veale, following a mining accident in 1895.[15] Modeled and cast in silver by a London artist, it is serviceable but generic in comparison to the finely wrought, personalized masks recorded in Nicholls's photographs. Nevertheless, Veale's gratitude is evident in an article published in the dental magazine *Ash's "Quarterly Circular"* in 1896, which includes the following testimonial from the patient:

> Not the least part of my trouble since recovery has been the necessity for wearing a heavy veil. I am thankful to say this is no longer needed, for by the kindness of two gentlemen who became interested in me (Mr Brock, dentist, and Mr Hudson, artist), an apparatus has been constructed which enables me to speak distinctly, to eat, drink, and smoke with comfort, and to appear in public without attracting attention.[16]

Plates and artificial noses were also worn by women whose faces had been disfigured by tuberculosis, lupus, syphilis, or smallpox. As we saw in the

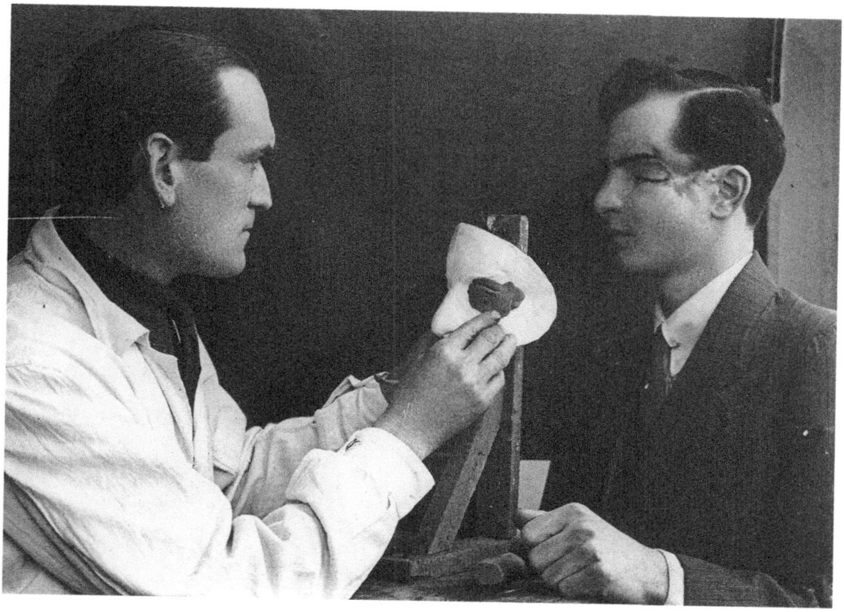

Fig. 29. Horace Nicholls, Captain Derwent Wood, R.A., who moulds the plates. Imperial War Museum, Q.30.456. (Photograph courtesy of the Imperial War Museum, London.)

last chapter, the disfigured face of war often resembled the physiognomy of disease, particularly in cases where the nose was damaged or missing. The difference was that the face of war was definitively male, whereas disease—particularly diseases, like syphilis, associated with moral degeneration and aberrant sexuality—often assumed a feminine guise in the Victorian imagination. One of the most dedicated chroniclers of the Victorian "monstrous feminine" was Arthur Munby (1828–1910), a London civil servant who compulsively watched, drew, photographed, and wrote about working-class women's bodies.[17] Munby eventually married Hannah Culwick, a domestic servant he met in 1854, and his obsession with her is the subject of Barry Reay's compelling book *Watching Hannah.* Another young woman to catch Munby's eye was Mary Anne Bell, who was eighteen and living in London when she first made an appearance in his diary. Disfigured by cancer as a child, she was left with a hole "the size of a sixpence" where her nose had been. Recalling their conversation in his journal, Munby wrote:

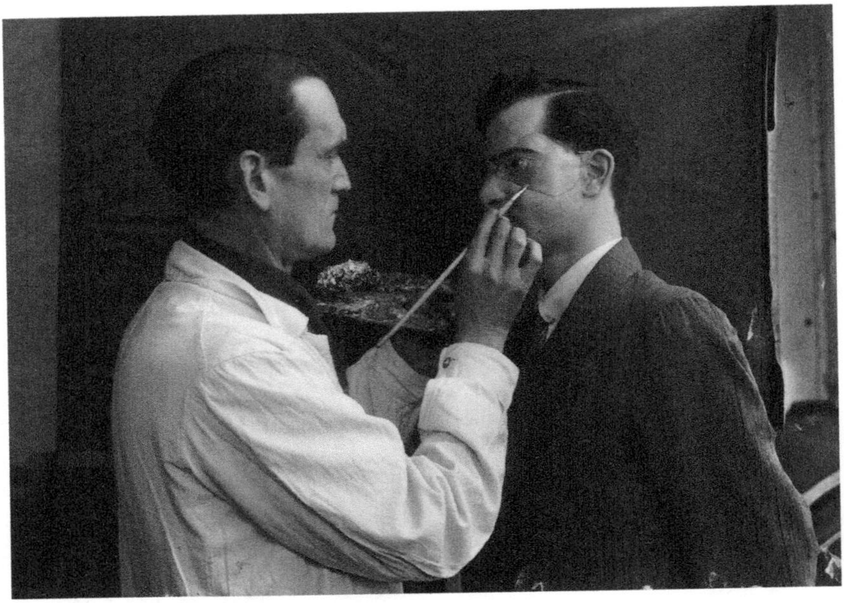

Fig. 30. Horace Nicholls, Painting the plate. Imperial War Museum, Q.30.457. (Photograph courtesy of the Imperial War Museum, London.)

> "Well Mary, your face looks quite nice now"—"Yes Sir it's a deal better, if only I get a nose put on"—"And when you've got a nose, what will you do?" "Well Sir, when I've got my nose, I think I shall go into service." "How? But won't they find out that you've got a false nose?" "No Sir, I expect not—they won't see the joining. My nose will be fastened on with a hook, and I can take it off when I like."[18]

Prosthetic noses had been made for centuries: Henry Wellcome collected half a dozen examples, carved out of ivory or cast and silver plated, along with a late eighteenth-century drawing of a man with an artificial nose (figures 34 and 35). Some three hundred years earlier, the French surgeon Ambroise Paré (ca. 1510–90) had compared the results of rhinoplasty and external prostheses. The story he recounts in his treatise on reparative surgery concerns the Cadet of Saint Thoan: a gentleman whose silver nose has long been a source of great amusement among his friends.[19] Hearing of a "master remaker of lost noses" in Italy, the cadet goes to find him and, in time, returns with a nose that everyone agrees is a great improvement. "Nevertheless," reflects Paré:

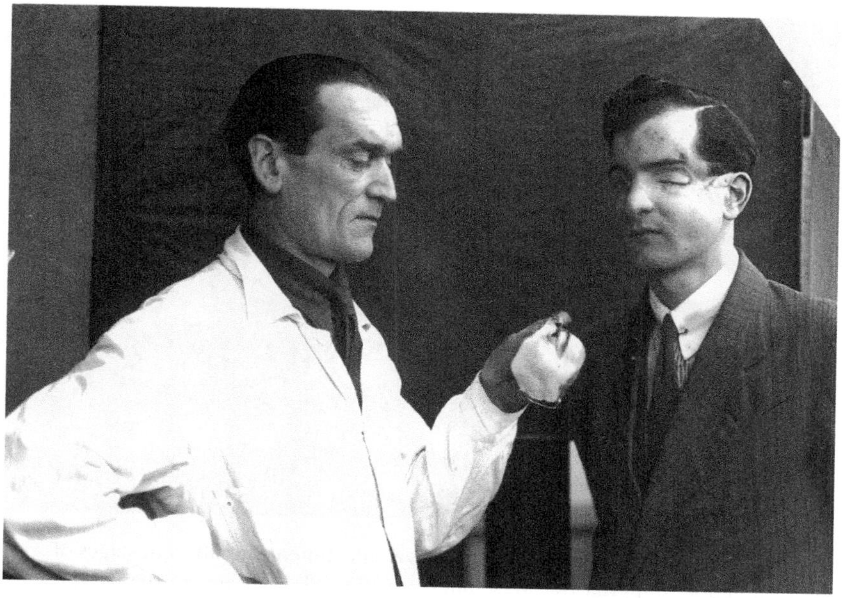

Fig. 31. Horace Nicholls, Examining the finished plate. Imperial War Museum, Q.30.458. (Photograph courtesy of the Imperial War Museum, London.)

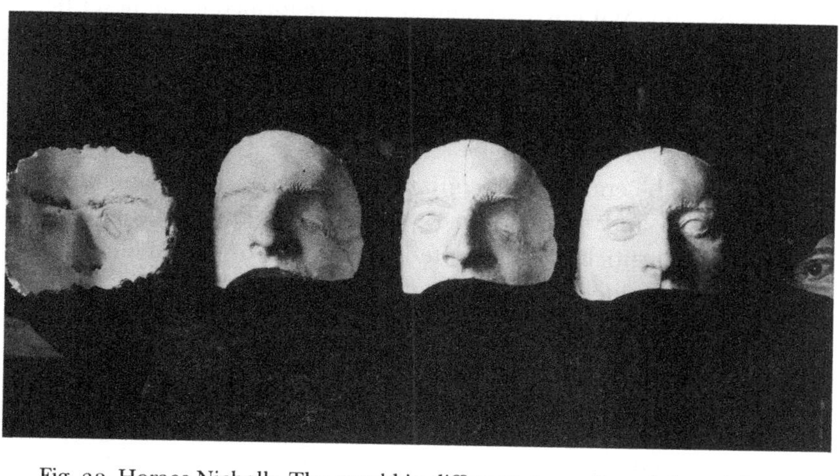

Fig. 32. Horace Nicholls, The mould in different stages. From left to right the mask mould, the mask cast, the cast with the good eye restored, the plate moulded, and the finished plate attachment. Imperial War Museum, Q.30.459. (Photograph courtesy of the Imperial War Museum, London.)

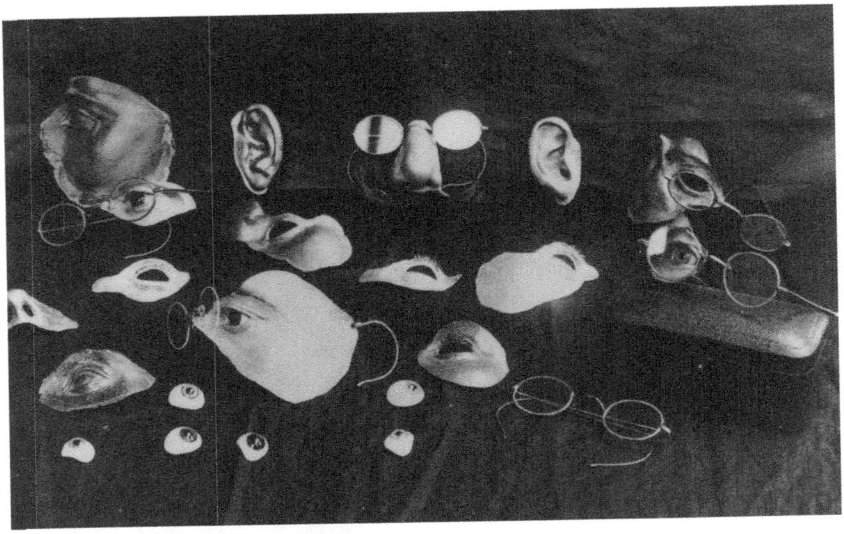

Fig. 33. Horace Nicholls, Various plates & attachments in different stages of completion. Imperial War Museum, Q.30.460. (Photograph courtesy of the Imperial War Museum, London.)

> It seems to me very difficult and burdensome to the patient. . . . [I]n addition, this flesh is not the same quality nor similar to that of the nose, and even when agglutinated and re-formed it can never be of the same shape and colour as that which was formerly in the place of the lost nose: likewise the openings of the nostrils can never be as they were originally.[20]

Paré's sixteenth-century text contains illustrations of enameled eyes, prosthetic ears and noses (figure 36), palatal obturators, mechanical limbs, and an artificial penis crafted from wood or tin. Made of gold, silver, paper, or glued linen cloths, his noses were "coloured, counterfeited and made both of fashion, figure and bigness, that [they] may as aptly as is possible resemble the natural nose."[21] Nicholls and Muir were most likely unaware of this longer history of facial repair, although they may have seen masks like William Veale's or noses like the one Mary Bell dreamed of. And they would certainly have been attuned to the stigma of the missing nose, of which Gaston Leroux's *Phantom of the Opera*—translated into English in 1911—is the most famous expression. The Phantom has several disguises, including a "long, thin, and transparent" nose and another made of pasteboard, with a moustache attached to it, which he wears when he has to venture out in public.[22]

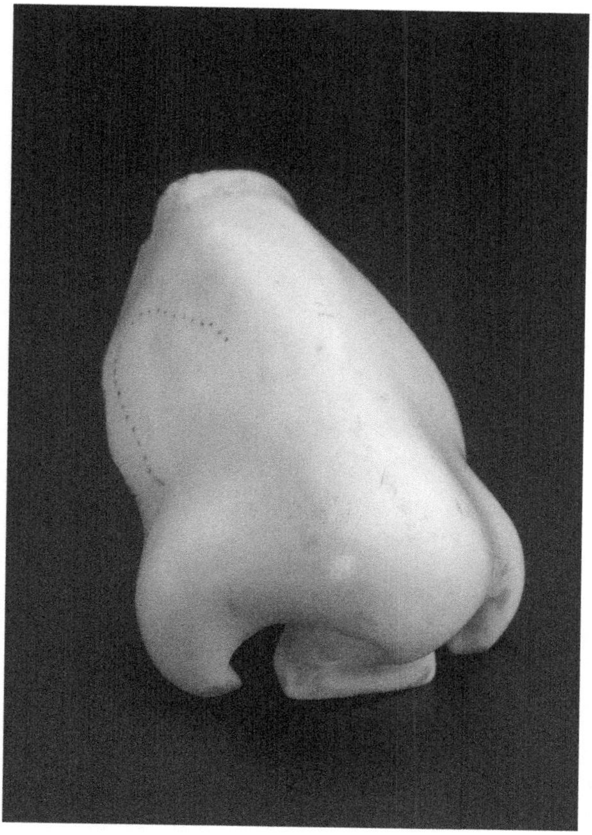

Fig. 34. Prosthetic nose carved from a single piece of ivory, Europe, 1701–1800. There are no holes for ties, suggesting that the nose was fixed directly to the face. Wellcome Library, London.

Nicholls presumably kept working notes, but no written record of the photographs of Derwent Wood has survived, apart from the original captions. The same year, however, Ward Muir—also an orderly at the Third London General—wrote *The Happy Hospital*, an intimate account of the hospital and its patients. Apart from being a prolific writer and a corporal in the RAMC, Muir was a passionate amateur photographer. Excerpts from *The Happy Hospital* appeared in the *Spectator*, *Nineteenth Century*, *Country Life*, the *Daily News*, and the *New Statesman*, and Muir also edited *Happy—Though Wounded*, a fund-raising compilation of stories, poems, anecdotes, and artwork from the hospital *Gazette*. In the final chapter of the book we find a passage that resembles Nicholls's photographs to an uncanny degree, as though the two men, photographer and writer, were observing the same event (there is no mention of Nicholls in Muir's account). "Let me take you into the Masks for Facial Disfigurements Department," Muir begins:

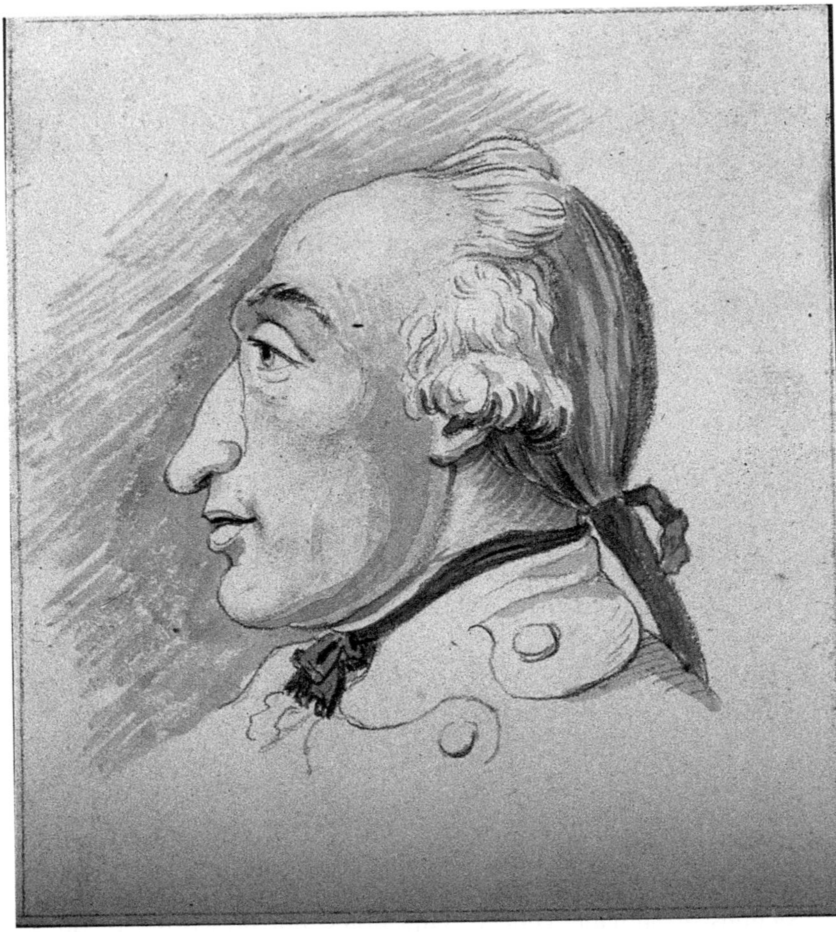

Fig. 35. A man with an artificial nose. Pencil drawing with wash, ca. 1791. From the first English version of J. C. Lavater's *Essays on Physiognomy* (1789–98). The subject of the portrait, Lavater explains, lost his nose in an accident. The illustration demonstrates the "homogeneousness" of the face: "a long descending nose like this alone could have fitted him: this progression was the only true one, every other would have been incongruous." Wellcome Library, London.

The room, divided by a partition, is half a workshop and half a studio. In the workshop we encounter a Lance-Corporal who, as a civilian, was a sculptor's moulder by trade. . . . He presides over a bench, a litter of esoteric implements, a bag of plaster of Paris, some plasticine, a sink, and a geyser for hot water. In the studio we find the sculptor (but a sculptor attired as a Captain of the British Army): and likewise some

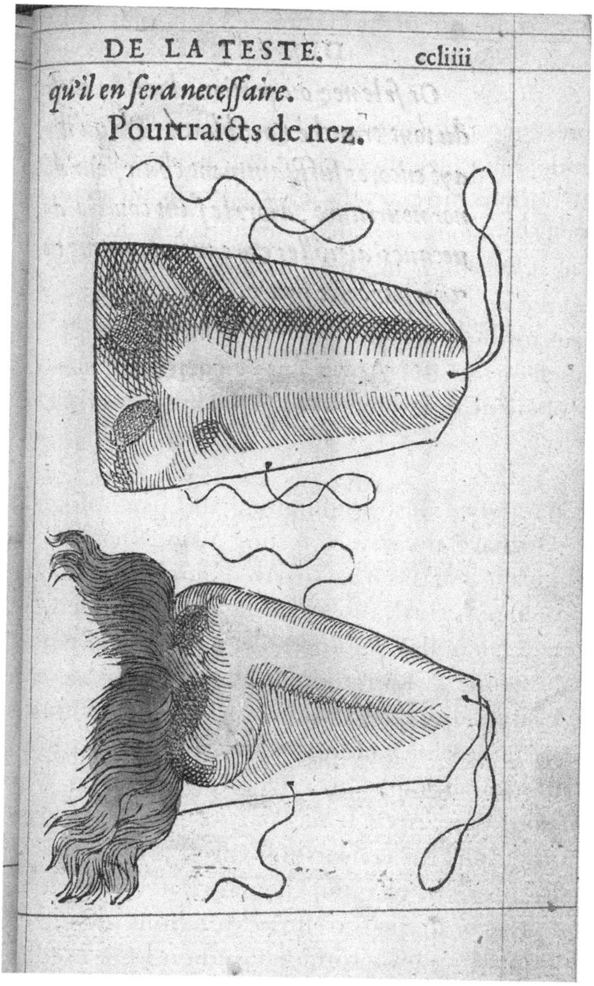

Fig. 36. Hand-colored illustration of a prosthetic nose. From Ambroise Paré, *La methode curative des playes, et fractures de la teste humaine*, 1561. Wellcome Library, London.

> of his odd sculptures, frail little painted bits of human visages, some with neat moustaches and a pair of spectacles attached to them; and, on the walls, a frieze of souvenirs in the shape of casts of those same visages, with photographs of their owners in the flesh—the "before" and "after" records which so promptly demolish the criticisms of the theorising objector.[23]

Muir relates the successive stages of casting and modeling much as Nicholls depicts them, noting the "unforeseen value" of preinjury portrait photographs as reference material, the meticulous re-creation of an eye, eyebrow, and eyelashes, and the use of spectacles or spirit gum to hold the finished mask in place. "It is difficult," he writes,

> to convey a fair impression of the extraordinary, thousandth-of-an-inch sort of correctitude with which these membrane-like but strong metal masks adhere to the face and cover the grisly gap beneath them. At a slight distance, so harmonious are both the molding and the tinting, it is impossible to detect the join where the live skin of cheek or nose leaves off and the imitation complexion of the mask begins. Figure what this means for the patient! Instead of being a gargoyle, ashamed to show himself on the streets, he is almost a normal human being and can go anywhere unafraid—unafraid (a happy release!) of seeing others afraid.[24]

Derwent Wood, as we have seen, also highlighted the psychological benefits of the masks. We have no way of testing Wood's claims or Muir's speculations. While a few masks have survived, none of them are Wood's.[25] They were either not worn, discarded as the men aged, or buried with their owners.[26] Nicholls's photographs bring us no closer to the interior lives of these men, whose thoughts and feelings we can only guess at. As artful historical documents then, what can Nicholls's photographs tell us? It is impossible to answer this question without first establishing what the photographs are, if not propaganda. Why were they taken? How were they used? It was part of Nicholls's brief to submit all of his photographs for censorship. Given the culture of aversion described in the previous chapter, they were never likely to appear in the illustrated press or in the traveling exhibitions organized by Wellington House.[27] Photographs of wounded soldiers were used in wartime propaganda, but as Sanders and Taylor observe, the pictures were typically "stage-managed" so as to suggest "fatigue being accompanied by cheerfulness," and wounds were invariably freshly dressed.[28]

Facial injury was very occasionally depicted in the illustrated papers, but always in the context of industrious convalescence, and the visibly disfigured face is rarely shown. Nicholls's photographs come closer to the fantasy of perfect repair than other images of facial casualties—the medical case photographs, for example, or Henry Tonks's portraits of facially injured soldiers before and after surgery. The two men who appear in the IWM albums are self-composed, their wounds less horrific than many of those on record, but still it is hard to imagine them serving as propaganda. The photographs are pensive rather than reassuring, capturing the loss alluded to in written accounts as well as the sculptor's skill; a loss that goes to the core of what it is to be recognizable, and even human. Nicholls's own son had enlisted under age, and was killed on the western front in April 1917.[1] It is hard not to see these images as personal meditations on the fragility of life and the inescapable presence of death. They record the hope of reconstruction and—at the same time—its impossibility. The unnamed patient is painstakingly restored, his blind eye opened with a stroke of the paintbrush, but in the end—when we are shown Wood examining the finished plate—it is the exquisite artificiality of the mask one is drawn to, the absence of life, for the mask replicates a face that no longer exists.

Nicholls had an instinct for visual storytelling, a skill he had honed as a freelance photographer, self-publicist, and raconteur. In her biography of Nicholls, Gail Buckland paints a vivid picture of him as minor celebrity on the lantern slide circuit in late Victorian and Edwardian England, entertaining and educating audiences from London to Dundee with his eyewitness account of the Boer War. "Fresh from the Front," for example, toured the country in the winter and spring of 1900, raising a profit for the Lord Mayor's War Fund as well as supplementing Nicholls's comfortable middle-class income.[29] His professional success depended largely on finding an angle and treatment that would give him the edge over the competition. As Buckland observes, he "set out to make 'studies,' as they were then called—pictures that people were expected to look at carefully, not just glance at."[30] The standard format would be a full-page or even double-page feature, with smaller inserts surrounding a central image, for which Nicholls would charge between ten shillings and eight pence (for reproductions up to six inches by four inches) and twenty-one shillings (up to nine inches by six inches). Newspapers and magazines often reserved space for reproducing works of art, and that is where Nicholls aimed to place his photographs.[31]

Although he had less freedom to choose his subject matter during the 1914–18 war—and did not have to worry about selling his work—we see Nicholls making similar narrative and aesthetic choices as he recounts the daily routine of a factory worker, the transformation of a new recruit, or the reconstruction of a damaged face.[32] In a letter to Ivor Nicholson in September 1916, he wrote: "The chief aim of my work in photography is pictorial effect in preference to photographing anything and everything."[33] Whatever else they might be, the "Repairing war's ravages" pictures were conceived as a new kind of photojournalism, blending "pictorial effect" with topical interest.

The entwined histories of photojournalism and propaganda in World War I Britain go some of the way toward explaining Nicholls's output, but they do not account for the vast number of photographs that remained unseen by the public. Are we to suppose that the weighty albums that line the shelves at the Imperial War Museum are full of the failures—either too politically sensitive to serve as propaganda, or not artful enough for publication? At the end of the war, in December 1918, the Ministry of Information was transformed into the Imperial War Museum. Nicholls remained on staff, with responsibility for conserving all the photographic negatives in the ministry's possession, including his own twenty-three hundred negatives of the home front. When he retired fifteen years later, in 1932, *The Sunday Dispatch* announced that "The guardian of 100,000 photographic negatives at the Imperial War Museum and 100,000 memories of all parts of the world has retired."[34]

As part of this collection of "memories," what do Nicholls' World War I photographs have in common? We have looked at their social and institutional contexts, and the ways in which Nicholls exploits the aesthetic and narrative potential of his medium, but what is it that holds these objects together as an archive? The visual anthropologist and historian Elizabeth Edwards cautions that we need to "think serially" when approaching photographic archives. Sometimes an archive is united by the photographer's or commissioner's intention; sometimes the collector's eye, or the archivist's cataloging system. The unifying principle might be subject matter or style, or the material and epistemological practices of mounting, storing, and labeling. Nicholls's photographs of the home front are, to borrow Edwards's phrase, "linked visual events"—even if they were also meant to be viewed individually, attentively, as works of art.[35]

Might the home front photographs have been commissioned not (or not only) as wartime propaganda, but as a historical record and official "memory"? There is nothing in Nicholls's correspondence with Wellington House to provide a definitive answer to this question, but Ivor Nicholson and his colleagues must have been familiar with the contemporary idea of the "camera as historian." This was the title of a handbook published in May 1916 for use by members of the burgeoning Photographic Record Societies across the UK.[36] Nicholls's approach was, as we have seen, quite unlike the "straightforward and ordered" methods advocated by the photographic survey movement.[37] The difference can be seen most clearly in the labels, which betray none of the epistemological "anxiety" Edwards attributes to the librarians, archivists, and photographers involved with the survey movement for whom accuracy, storage, and retrievability were pressing concerns.[38] Nicholls clearly was not burdened by the same standards of exactitude and objectivity. His captions omit factual details like dates, places, and names. They communicate narrative intention rather than scientific aspiration. And yet the sheer number, as well as the range and detail of his wartime output, is a legacy of the "encyclopedic turn" of the nineteenth century.[39] He was, wittingly or not, making history on behalf of the British government; and like every historical record, his was both personal and partial.

Paris

A second workshop for portrait masks opened in Paris in November 1917 under the supervision of the American Red Cross Bureau for Reeducation of the Mutilated. Its director, Anna Coleman Ladd (1878–1939), had completed her education in Paris and Rome, where she studied under Phillip Hale and Charles Grafly. By 1915 she was married to an eminent Boston pediatrician, Maynard Ladd, and had established a name for herself as a sculptor and socialite, with portrait commissions from the likes of Anna Pavlova, Princess Borghese, and the actress Eleanor Duse. When the United States entered the war in the spring of 1917, Ladd's husband assumed responsibility for the Children's Bureau for the American Red Cross in Toul. The suggestion that she might go to France herself and make portrait masks for the mutilated seems to have come from the English art critic Lewis Hind, who mentioned Derwent Wood's initiative during a visit to Ladd's studio in Massachusetts.[40] In a letter referring to their conversation, Hind expresses his confidence that, should she go to Europe, her "talents as a sculptor and modeller would be of immense help in this service to humanity."[41]

By Christmas she was installed in a large fifth-floor artist's studio in the Latin Quarter. Among Ladd's papers in the Archives of American Art are sepia prints of a bright, high-ceilinged room decorated with posters, flowers, and an American flag. "American Red Cross, Place de la Concorde" is stamped on the back of the photographs.[42] Most are before-and-after portraits (for example, figures 37 and 38), some taken in front of an improvised black curtain. One wall of the studio is hung with casts of wounded faces, arranged in rows with eyes shut tight like an array of death masks. Some of the finished plates are displayed on a makeshift tablecloth; a vase of lilies and a small figurine of a woman complete the

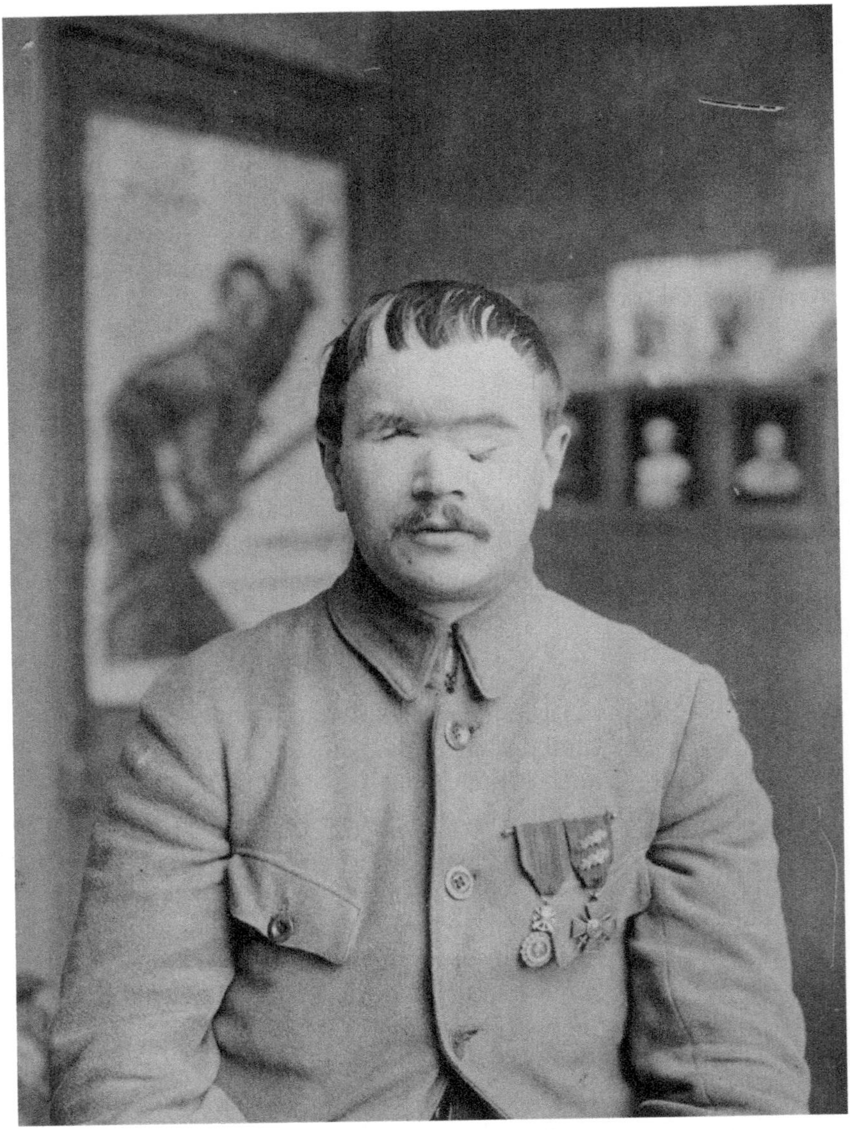

Fig. 37. World War I soldier facial reconstruction documentation photograph before fitting with mask, ca. 1918 / American Red Cross, photographer: photographic print: b&w; 17 × 13 cm. Anna Coleman Ladd papers, ca. 1881–1950, Archives of American Art, Smithsonian Institution.

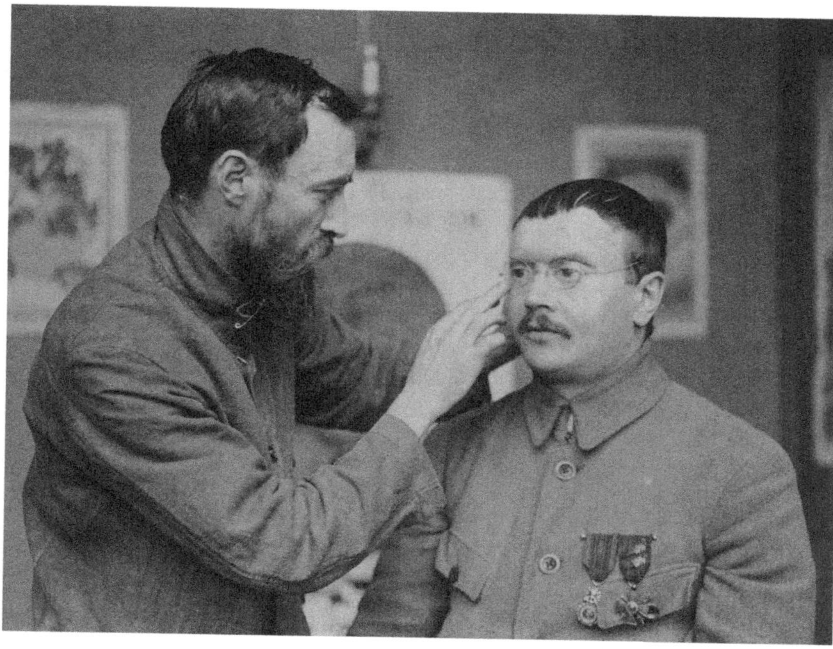

Fig. 38. World War I soldier facial reconstruction documentation photograph of a fitting, ca. 1918 / American Red Cross, photographer: photographic print: b&w; 11 × 17 cm. Anna Coleman Ladd papers, ca. 1881–1950, Archives of American Art, Smithsonian Institution.

ensemble (figure 39). While the medical subject matter of the casts is novel, plaster replicas of legs, arms, feet, and hands—displayed on walls or lined up on bookshelves—were a common sight in artists' studios of the time and served as "*aide-memoires* or models in their own creative practice."[43] Auguste Rodin is known to have cast a dressing gown in 1897 as a study for his statue of Balzac; other artists obtained casts from dealers, or commissioned specialist casters.[44]

Jane Poupelet (1874–1932), who had trained in Rodin's circle and exhibited at the Paris Salon of 1904, oversaw the day-to-day running of the studio while Ladd traveled to military hospitals across France to find suitable patients.[45] One of Poupelet's sculptures—a little bronze rabbit—is visible on a shelf in several of the photographs.[46] Other staff included the sculptor Robert Wlérick, a friend of Poupelet, and Diana Blair, from the Harvard Medical Laboratory.[47] In the final year of the war, the studio produced sixty-five masks for French and American servicemen and two for female civilians who had suffered facial burns during a bom-

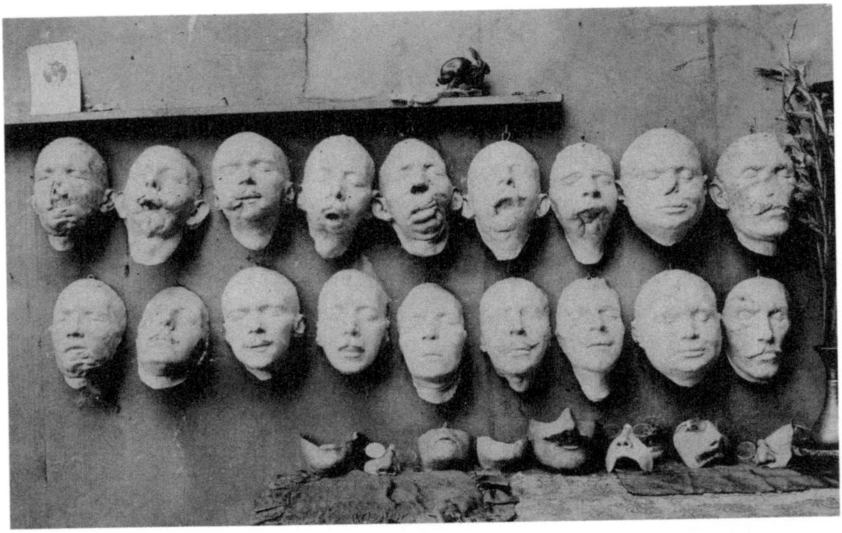

Fig. 39. World War I soldier facial reconstruction casts and masks, ca. 1918 / American Red Cross, photographer: photographic print: silver gelatin; b&w; 12 × 17 cm. Anna Coleman Ladd papers, ca. 1881–1950, Archives of American Art, Smithsonian Institution.

bardment.[48] Ladd returned to the United States in January 1919, and in October that year the Studio for Portrait Masks moved to new premises in the Hospital du Val-de-Grâce. Poupelet stayed on until 1920, overseeing the making of a further 153 masks.[49]

In a silent film commissioned by the American Red Cross, the studio at 70 Rue Notre Dame des Champs comes to life. Ladd walks briskly along the street, through a cast iron gate into a courtyard hung with ivy. In the studio, three uniformed *mutilés* are having new features sculpted, painted, and fitted. The man nearest the camera takes the cigarette from his mouth, reaches behind his ear and, with a smile, removes his chin. His compatriots are just as easy in the company of Ladd's assistants, nodding and chatting while the sculptors make adjustments. A plaster ear is wired up to a battery and lowered into what looks like a soup tureen: after several days in this bath of copper sulfate, a thin metal film will have been deposited on the surface. The social intimacy and conviviality revealed in (and no doubt performed for) the camera is conspicuously different from the deep unease that pervades Ward Muir's account, or the still melancholy of Nicholls's photographs. In Paris, the Studio for

Portrait Masks evidently served a social as well as therapeutic function. There was a regular Tuesday tea, and at any one time there might be half a dozen visitors: the men we see in the photographs and film, but also surgeons and interested members of the public.[50] As Ladd recollected:

> Oftentimes these *poilus* would come in with gifts of flowers for the studio. We always tried to keep the place cheerful and frequently had the boys sitting around playing games. The blind ones played dominoes and the others checkers. We served them chocolates, cigarettes and their favorite *vin blanc*, and I defy anyone to find a happier group than was there assembled in that Parisian studio. They were never treated as though anything were the matter with them. We laughed with them and helped them to forget. That is what they longed for and deeply appreciated.[51]

Unlike staff at a military hospital—whose priority was to return the wounded to active service—Ladd and Poupelet saw their job as humanitarian: enabling the mutilated to return to civilian and domestic life.[52] A second film, now lost, narrated the homecoming of a *mutilé* and his daughter's failure to recognize him. With a portrait mask to cover his disfigurement, he is able to return, no longer a stranger to his family.[53] "So lifelike and personal were the masks," Ladd claimed, that children frequently cried out, "Here comes papa!"[54] Back in the United States, she embarked on a series of public lectures about her work in France. Articles in magazines and the Sunday papers quoted from the letters of gratitude sent by her "boys" and reproduced photographs from her personal album. The *Philadelphia Press* clipping reproduced in figure 40 includes the following excerpt from a letter:

> I am so happy again . . . that I not only dare to go home, but I am to have a home of my own. My fiancée pronounced me "*tres bien*" and does not shrink from me in repulsion, as she has a perfect right to do. Thanks to you and to splendid America.[55]

American newspaper editors were clearly less constrained than their British counterparts when it came to printing photographs of disfigured veterans: the war was over; it was a good story (featuring French *poilus* rather than mutilated Americans), and Ladd's enthusiasm was unshakeable. She even traveled with a selection of masks: a macabre variation on

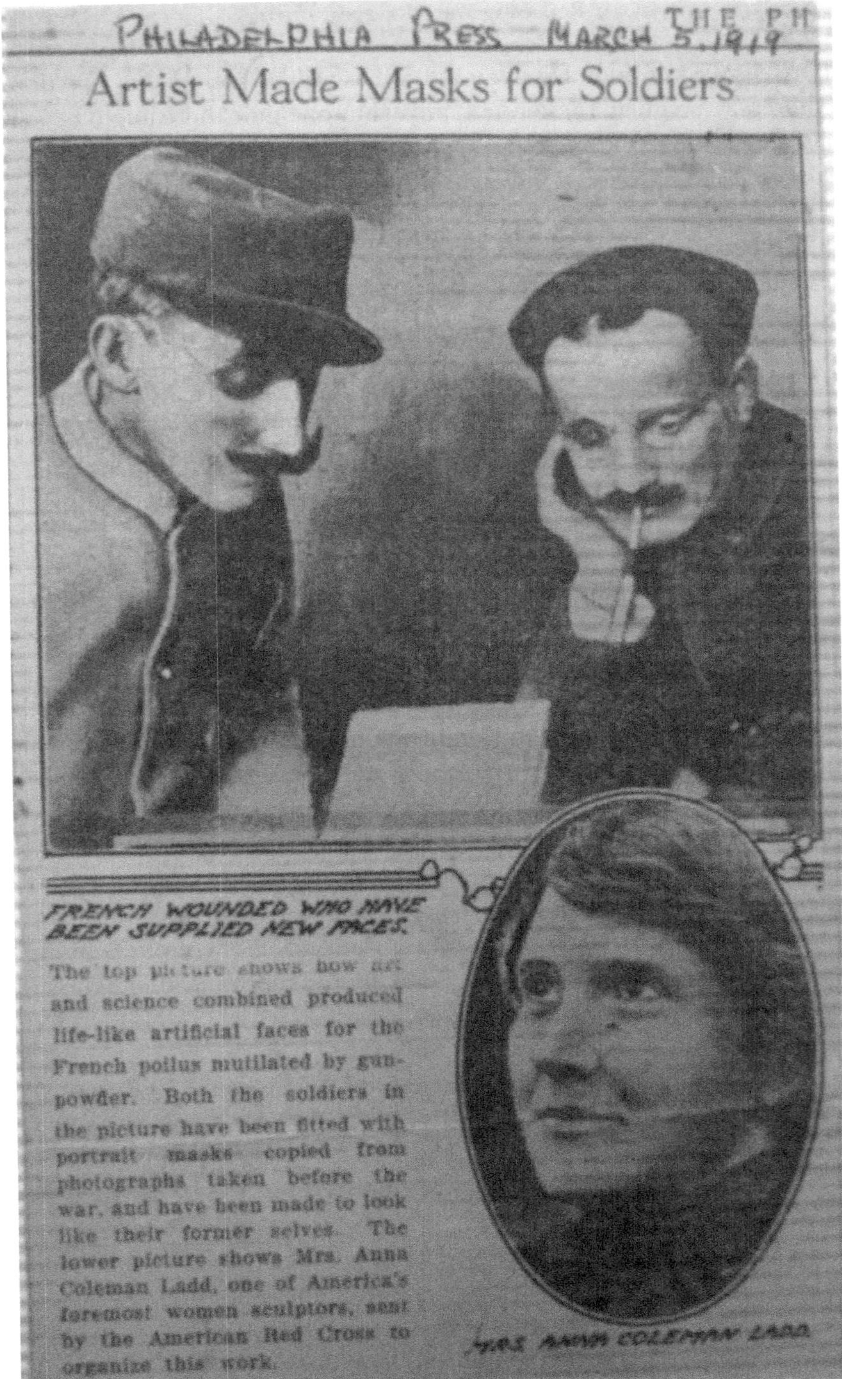

THE PH

Philadelphia Press March 5, 1919

Artist Made Masks for Soldiers

FRENCH WOUNDED WHO HAVE BEEN SUPPLIED NEW FACES.

The top picture shows how art and science combined produced life-like artificial faces for the French poilus mutilated by gunpowder. Both the soldiers in the picture have been fitted with portrait masks copied from photographs taken before the war, and have been made to look like their former selves. The lower picture shows Mrs. Anna Coleman Ladd, one of America's foremost women sculptors, sent by the American Red Cross to organize this work.

MRS. ANNA COLEMAN LADD

Fig. 40. "Artist Made Masks for Soldiers," *Philadelphia Press*, March 5, 1919. Anna Coleman Ladd papers, ca. 1881–1950, Archives of American Art, Smithsonian Institution.

the nineteenth-century cult of the souvenir. Muriel Caswall, writing for the *Sunday Post*, remarked:

> I saw some of these copper features lying on her table at the Hotel Charlesgate, where [Ladd] and her husband are now staying, and the effect was truly startling. They looked for all the world like human noses and chins laid out for a cannibal's supper.[56]

To the extent that they hid what could not be shown, the bespoke masks produced by Francis Derwent Wood in London and Anna Coleman Ladd in Paris are consistent with the history of stigma and censorship charted in chapter 2. Like most artists of their generation, Wood and Ladd saw beauty and ugliness in moral terms. As David Lubin observes of Ladd, "She revered physical beauty and believed, with wholehearted conviction, that ugliness and deformity should be kept out of sight."[57] He concludes that "the portrait mask enterprise"—despite the noble intentions of those involved—was "one more officially sanctioned attempt to conceal war's brutality behind a false front."[58] Before we consider their significance as *portraits*, it is imperative that this act of concealment be understood in social as well as ideological and aesthetic terms.

One of the critical factors in the social management of stigma, according to Goffman, is the extent to which the stigmatizing condition "interferes with the flow of interaction."[59] He gives the example of a blind person with a white cane. Although the cane is conspicuous and functions as a "stigma symbol," it doesn't disrupt social communication; however, "The blind person's failure to direct his face to the eyes of his co-participants is an event that repeatedly violates communication etiquette and repeatedly disrupts the feedback mechanics of spoken interaction."[60] Goffman distinguishes between attributes, such as the white cane, that are evident—there is no chance of passing as a sighted person—and those that are "obtrusive." It is, I would suggest, the perceived "obtrusiveness" of facial disfigurement—and not just its visibility—that the masks ameliorate.

A mask can be a likeness; it can be a disguise; but the term is also used to mean "a covering for all or part of the face."[61] "Many of those who rarely try to pass," notes Goffman, "routinely try to cover."[62] Dark glasses can signify (and draw attention to) visual impairment, while at the same time concealing any facial disfigurement: they reveal "unsightedness while concealing unsightliness."[63] In exactly the same way, a mask might signify disfigurement (it is a "stigma symbol" in Goffman's terms)

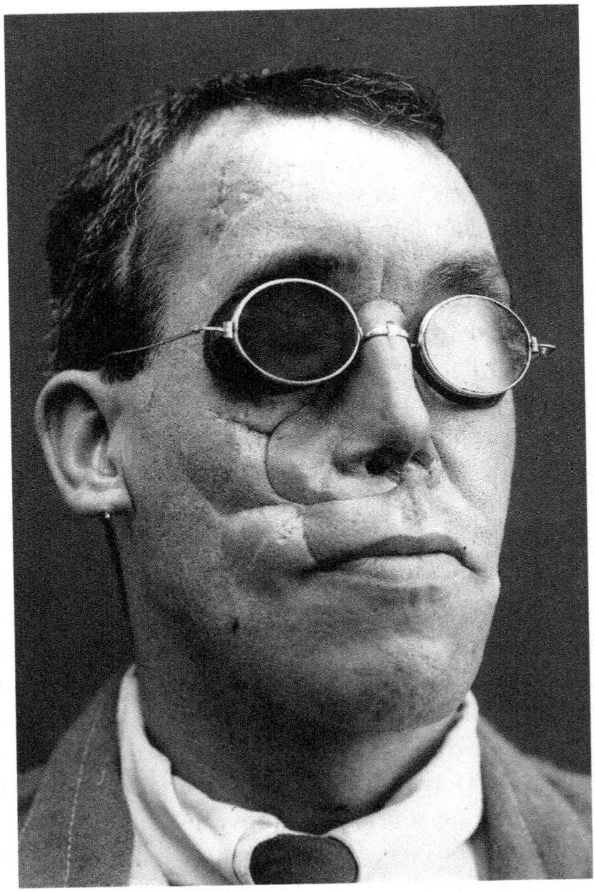

Fig. 41. Photograph of rifleman E. Moss from MS0513/1/1/ID1477. From the Archives of the Royal College of Surgeons of England.

while lessening the "obtrusiveness" of the severely disfigured face. The masks produced by Wood and Ladd could never replicate the warmth and expressive range of a human face, but they could hide the "dreadful abyss" of raw being and restore a conventional semblance of humanity.[64] Wearing a plate or mask—however crude or unconvincing—was part of a social contract not to offend, not to be obtrusive. I will spare you the sight of my face, the mask declares.

For Rifleman Moss (figures 41 and 42), dark glasses and a prosthetic nose (not by Wood in this instance) conceal the injury documented in figure 42. He would hardly have been inconspicuous, but as his surgeon Gillies later remarked, "Fitted with an external prosthesis, at least he was presentable enough to be a blind man."[65]

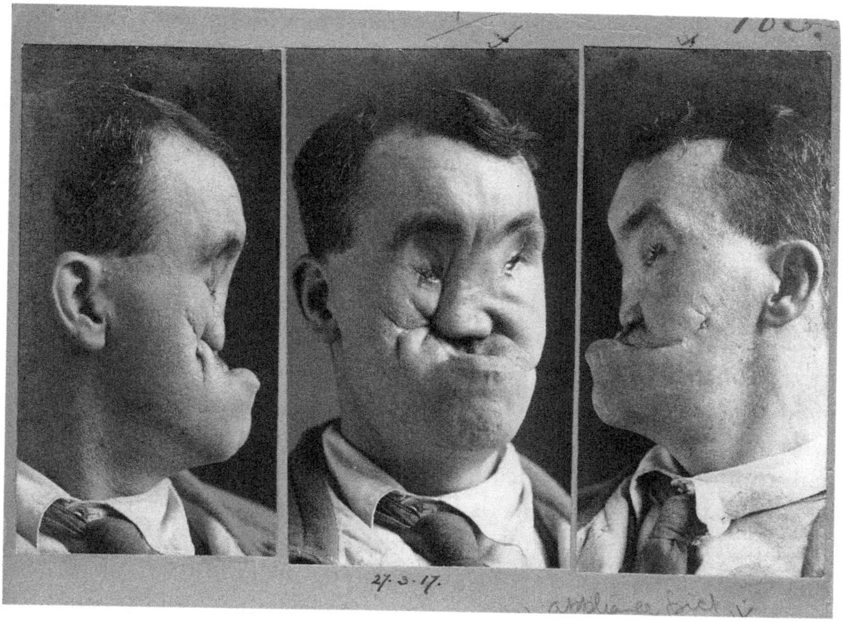

Fig. 42. Photographs of E. Moss from MS0513/1/1/ID1477. From the Archives of the Royal College of Surgeons of England.

The Cast Portrait

Anna Ladd was awarded the Legion of Honor in 1933: an occasion that was marked by an illustrated feature in the *St. Louis Post-Dispatch* Sunday magazine. Her aim, she explained to her interlocutor, had not simply been "to provide a man a mask to hide his awful mutilation, but to put in that mask part of the man himself—that is, the man he had been before tragedy intervened."[66] On the one hand, Ladd implies, the masks served to conceal their wearers' true condition (and, by extension, the horror of war); on the other, they embodied something essential ("part of the man himself") that had been irreparably damaged. There is a paradox here. The mask is a condoned deception (as theatrical masks have always been); and yet its greatest virtue is its authenticity. Interestingly, cosmetic surgery is often debated today in exactly these terms. It is seen both as a masquerade (in which the surgically altered face takes on the appearance and function of a theatrical mask) *and* as a means of rejuvenation or repair in which the "natural" body is at best latent and provisional:

realized by the surgeon and the consumer. There is, however, a very specific sense in which the masks produced by Ladd and Wood *contained* their subjects, and it has more to do with the nineteenth-century fashion for cast portraits than the emerging practice of aesthetic surgery in early twentieth-century Britain and America. The final part of this chapter considers the history and conceptual legacy of the life mask as a form of likeness that literally contained—in the form of a physical impression—its subject.

According to Pliny the Elder (AD 23–79), life casting was invented by the ancient Greek sculptor Lysistratus, whose likenesses were especially prized for their accuracy.[67] Revived during the Italian Renaissance, the technique was famously practiced by the fifteenth-century Florentine artist (and Leonardo's teacher) Andrea del Verocchio, who used it to make both life masks and death masks.[68] But the earliest practical guide to casting the human figure is Cennino Cennini's late fourteenth- or early fifteenth-century handbook *Il Libro Dell'Arte*, which offers detailed advice on casting an "effigy or physiognomy" from life. The person to be cast must lie flat on a table or bench, he explains, while an iron collar is fastened around the face. Have a goldsmith make little silver or brass breathing tubes that will fit in the nostrils, Cennini suggests: the wet plaster can then be safely poured onto the face until it is a finger's depth from the tip of the nose and left to set. "And bear in mind," he adds, "that if this person whom you are casting is very important, as in the case of lords, kings, popes, emperors, you mix this plaster with tepid rose water; and for other people any tepid spring or well or river water is good enough."[69]

Life and death masks were made for commemorative purposes well into the twentieth century. The Slade School archives, for example, contain a death mask of Henry Tonks, probably made by two of his former students, William Coldstream and Walter Thomas Monnington, shortly after the artist's death in 1937.[70] Facial casts were used as the basis of portrait busts, often posthumously, but they were also displayed in domestic settings as mementos of loved ones, both living and dead. More affordable than carved or modeled likenesses, cast portraits in plaster, clay, or wax—especially those of the living face—could preserve "the exact similitude of every feature."[71] Like the photographic portraits that eventually replaced them, life masks are more than just accurate likenesses: they evoke the presence of their subjects in a particularly direct way. At close range, the caster's skill (or lack thereof) is tangible: the casts made by the nineteenth-century French sculptor Adolphe-Victor Geoffroy-

Dechaume perfectly reproduce his models' skin. You can see the goose bumps caused by the chill of liquid plaster on bare skin.[72] Rosalind Krauss defines the index as "that type of sign which arises as the physical manifestation of a cause, of which traces, imprints, and clues are examples."[73] Like photographs, cast portraits are indexical signs because we experience them as imprints or traces of an original rather than pictorial "representations." They *are* their subject matter in an ontological sense.

A good portrait, however, is expected to be more than a facsimile. For Rodin, "To copy nature faithfully is not the purpose of art. A life cast is the most accurate copy one can get, but it is lifeless, it lacks movement and eloquence, it does not say everything."[74] In order for a portrait to succeed—for it to be *eloquent*—the artist needed to "read behind the facial mask."[75] Ladd, who once claimed to have been instructed by Rodin,[76] would have been familiar with the idea of art as a product of imagination and understanding (an argument that was more frequently rehearsed in relation to photography). And like Rodin, her conception of portraiture was essentially psychological. In the absence of preinjury photographs, she resorted to established nonfacial signifiers of personality:

> In many cases I was able to work from photographs. But sometimes there were none. However, from a study of all the features of the man which indicate his character and personality—finger tips, ear lobes, and so on, and through chats with the victims and their friends, I was able in every case to give the mutilated, disheartened man back his personality, and his hopes, and ambitions.[77]

This chapter has focused on portrait masks, but the techniques of casting and modeling were also used to plan reconstructive facial surgery. Captain Holtzapffel, who was treated by Harold Gillies at the Ellerman Hospital in Regent's Park, described the "strange and uncomfortable process" of whole-face casting, "especially when the hardened plaster was pulled away giving one a most extraordinary feeling of being sucked all over one's face until the air got under at one corner when the whole thing lifted off easily." With the aid of photographs the plaster cast was "built up with wax into a portrait with a complete nose."[78] The sculptor in this case was Kathleen Scott (1878–1947), the widow of Captain Robert Falcon Scott, who had died returning from the South Pole in 1912. Kathleen, now Lady Scott, had studied with Henry Tonks at the Slade and completed her artistic training at the Académie Colarossi in Paris. Her wartime diaries record a meeting with Tonks in July 1916: "I spent the evening with Henry Tonks, who took me to the hospital, to the jaw-ward, to see his pastelles of facial wounds. One of a boy with his arm amputated and with a deep hole in his jaw is hauntingly beautiful" (figure 43).[79]

It was presumably Tonks who recommended her for the job of modeling and casting at the new Ellerman Hospital for officers in Regent's Park. "I think I will take that on," reads her entry for September 17, 1918. Her first patient was a man with no mouth. "They asked me if I could stand it, and I replied confidently that I could, and I did, but I was very unwell when the tension was over. This is what happens to me in emotion. I am very sick, I never cry."[80] A fortnight later the initial shock had subsided. Asked to model a new chin for a patient, Scott quips that it makes her feel "terribly like God, the creator," and on November 4—after she has spent the day working on "a man with a wonderful face and no nose"—she reflects on the resemblance of these war-damaged faces to classical Greco-Roman statues. "These men with no noses," she writes, "are very beautiful, like antique marbles."[81]

Like Anna Ladd, Derwent Wood and Jane Poupelet, Kathleen Scott's artistic training was based largely on the study of the antique, which usually meant drawing plaster casts of classical sculptures and sculptural fragments in a studio. Casts of specific poses and parts of the body taken from live models were gradually incorporated into this didactic tradition in the nineteenth century.[82] By likening the ruins of classical antiquity to the corporeal ravages of war, Scott—like Tonks—was able to respond to facial injury on an aesthetic level. But the casts displayed in rows in Ladd's studio and Wood's tell another story. From about 1840, scientists had used casts, in wax or plaster, to record and classify aspects of both the natural world and human culture. If the value of the cast portrait is its capacity to evoke an individual, the new disciplines of criminology, botany, zoology, dermatology, archaeology, and anthropology were concerned with taxonomies and types.

In 2002 the Henry Moore Foundation in Leeds organized an exhibition of historical and contemporary cast objects. The historical artifacts were selected from an earlier exhibition, *A Fleur de Peau,* held at the Musée d'Orsay in Paris. Sculptures by Rodin, Alexandre Falguière, and Geoffroy-Dechaume were juxtaposed with nineteenth-century medical, anthropological, and botanical casts (the latter exquisitely represented by a clump of plaster mushrooms cast by the naturalist Jean-Baptiste Barla: one of a series of 674 mushroom compositions). Works by Duane Hanson, Robert Gober, Sarah Lucas, John De Andrea, Abigail Lane, Jordan Baseman, and Paul Thek demonstrated the variety of uses to which

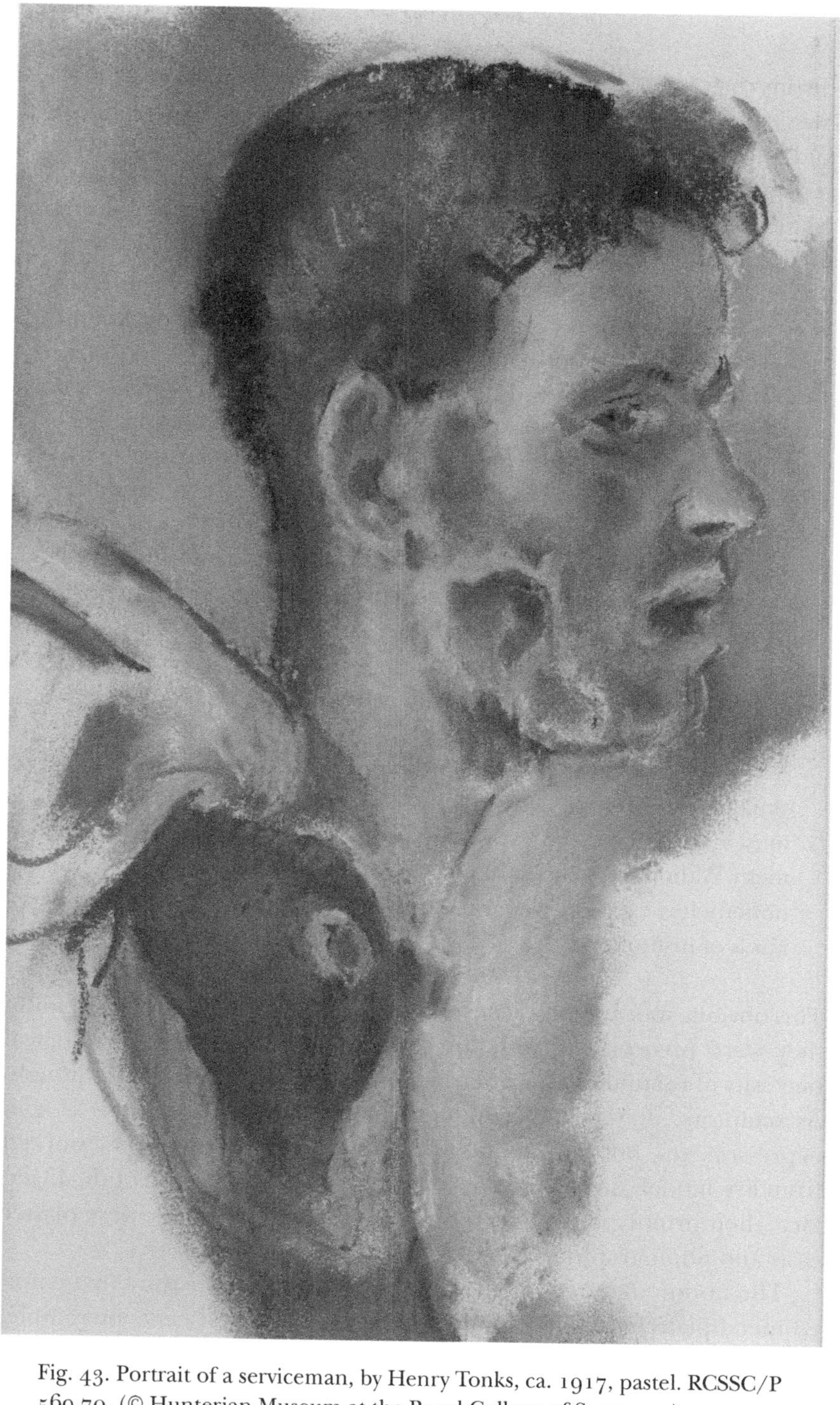

Fig. 43. Portrait of a serviceman, by Henry Tonks, ca. 1917, pastel. RCSSC/P 569.70. (© Hunterian Museum at the Royal College of Surgeons.)

casting has been put since the 1980s. The Leeds exhibition—*Second Skin*—succeeded in foregrounding the strangeness of these aesthetic and scientific objects. For they clearly offered more than a guarantee of verisimilitude: Stephen Feeke, in his catalog essay, ventures that it is their "skin" that makes them "so arresting."[83] Cast in wax, resin, aluminum, plaster, lead, ice, or bronze, human skin is rendered uncanny. And displayed in an art gallery or museum, a figure or face cast from life "allows us to scrutinise a stranger, a celebrity, a naked body or a corporeal fragment to a degree not normally possible."[84]

Like the masks discussed in this chapter, the casts in *Second Skin* are at once seductive, fascinating, and faintly repellent: arresting, as Feeke points out, because they license our gaze, repellent because their very lifelikeness underscores the absence of life. Despite their intimacy and verisimilitude, these are deathly objects. Even at their most eloquent, portraits—even Rodin's—cannot speak, and a mask cannot blush or express surprise, no matter how faithfully it replicates a human face. Furthermore, we don't just have one face, as Goffman points out: we have many. The "disciplined ordering of personal front" is one of the ways we express our "aliveness" to others. He elaborates:

> A very evident means by which the individual shows himself to be situationally present is by appropriately controlling through facial muscles the shape and expression of the various parts of this instrument. Although this control may not be conscious to any extent, it is nonetheless exerted. We have party faces, funeral faces, and various kinds of institutional faces.[85]

This obvious shortcoming is never discussed by Wood or Ladd. No doubt they were preoccupied with the practical challenges and ideological necessity of rebuilding men. Maybe there is more to it than that, though. As sculptors, they would habitually have thought of the face as still: expressive, yes, but not mobile or animate. And although they worked from live models, matching the contours, tone, and texture of the living face, their prototypes, as they rebuilt the damaged features, were plaster casts and photographs.

The notion that one might take comfort or even pleasure in a painted metal plate held in place by ribbons or spectacles seems incredible, but it may have mattered that these fragmentary portraits were precious objects in their own right, like a bespoke hat or a valuable item of jewelry. (Is it significant that Ladd's studio commissioned a famous Parisian firm of jewelers, Christofle, to plate the copper masks in silver?)[86] Perhaps the physical discomfort of wearing the masks, their ergonomic flaws and "lack of animate realism" were a small price to pay for an appearance.[87] Self-fashioning, after all, is always about performance and persuasion, compromise and artifice. It necessarily involves a kind of "wizardry," as Wood admitted.[88] And of course the pursuit of beauty or normality very often involves physical discomfort. This modern understanding of the self as something mutable, a creation (or re-creation), also comes across—albeit silently—in the film of Ladd's studio, which blurs the line between prosthetic and aesthetic reconstruction (and makes me think of beauty parlors and hairdressers rather than artists' studios).

There are clearly no easy answers to the question of the meaning and function of these perplexing objects. We can agree that they express a humanitarian impulse; that they were an attempt to ameliorate both the horror of war and the personal stigma of the mutilated face. But we know almost nothing about the men whose photographs and handwritten letters are archived with Ladd's papers, and even less about Wood's patients. Whether they wore their masks or put them at the back of a cupboard probably depends on the degree to which the men themselves, and those around them, experienced their disfigurement as obtrusive. For stigma, as Goffman shows, is always relational. In France, where the veterans known as *Les Gueules cassées*—the "broken faces"—were represented at the signing of the Treaty of Versailles, the visibility of disfigurement was collectively managed. Their British counterparts, in comparison, were politically invisible and socially isolated. Even if they were never worn, however, the masks reveal something about way the war-damaged face was understood at the time: as a "metaphor for the unutterable," to quote Claudine Mitchell, but also as a psychological and social wound.[89] In the next chapter we will look at a very different aesthetic response to facial injury. Like the masks made by Wood and Ladd, Tonks's drawings are reparative in intent, but they reveal disfigurement in its beauty as well as its horror, rather than concealing it.

CHAPTER 4

Flesh Poems

When I first saw Henry Tonks's drawings of facially injured soldiers, I was struck by how difficult it would be to write about them.[1] It's not just that the subject matter is disturbing. From the disciplinary perspectives of both art history and medicine, they are perplexing images. Are they portraits? The drawings (there are seventy-five in total) were neither commissioned nor owned by the men who appear in them: a framed selection hung on the wall of Tonks's room at the Queen's Hospital (figure 44), and on these he has recorded the sitter's name. The rest are identifiable only by cross-referencing their injuries with the documents in the case files.[2] Are they a graphic record of new surgical techniques? Tonks, who was teaching drawing at the Slade School of Art when the war broke out, started out with Gillies making diagrammatic records of the operations.[3] Photographs, some in stereograph, were also taken of the patients pre-and postoperatively. What do the pastels add to this extensive visual archive, apart from color?

Aside from the matter of their documentary function, these slightly smaller-than-life studies confront us with questions of spectatorship. Seeing them alongside the surgeon's notes and case photographs, I felt like a voyeur: my curiosity and distaste were surely inappropriate responses. Tonks himself was uncomfortable with the public interest in his drawings of damaged faces. In correspondence with Wellington House, the government's propaganda unit, he says that in his opinion the pastels are "rather dreadful subjects for the public view."[4] This is the only reference

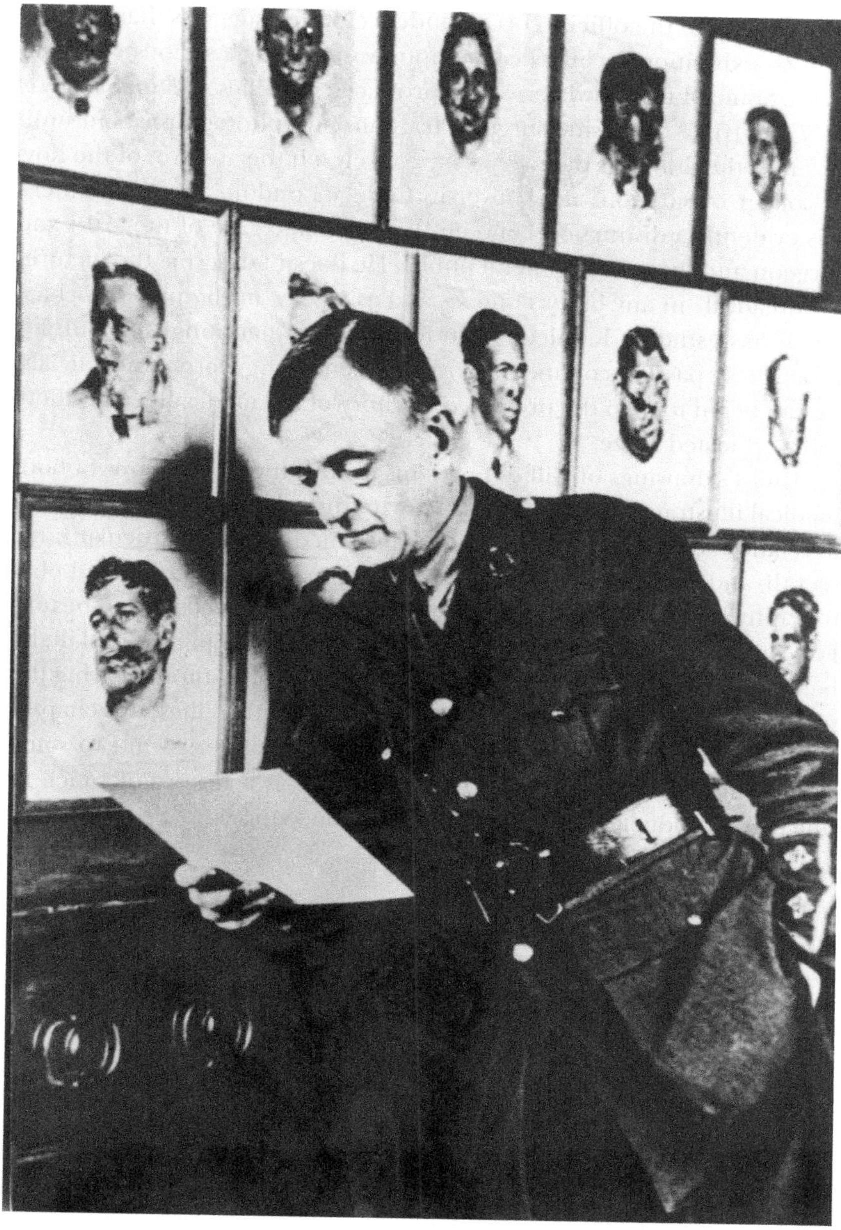

Fig. 44: Photograph of Henry Tonks in his room at the Queen's Hospital, Sidcup, 1917.

to the series in the official correspondence, which suggests that publication or exhibition for mass consumption was never a serious consideration. Some of the drawings were reproduced in Gillies's *Plastic Surgery of the Face* (1920) alongside surgical diagrams and photographs, but until recently, the drawings themselves have rarely left the archives of the Royal College of Surgeons and University College London.[5] For Tonks, there was evidently a distinction between the legitimate gaze of the artist and surgeon and that of the general public. He doesn't describe the pictures as "dreadful" in any other context, and as we saw in the previous chapter, Tonks's student Kathleen Scott found them "hauntingly beautiful."[6] From these passing comments, and the silence of government officials, we can begin to map the protected territory of the medically or aesthetically "educated" gaze.

Tonks's drawings of Gillies's patients disturb the conventions of both medical illustration and traditional portraiture. They are discussed here in relation to the visual cultures of modern medicine (in particular nineteenth- and twentieth-century traditions of medical illustration and photography) and the artist's own thoughts on artistic objectivity and beauty. For Tonks, good drawing was tactile: without this sensibility and skill, he believed, the draftsman's art was like playing a piano without hearing the notes. In light of Tonks's wartime collaboration with Gillies, this chapter also explores the hypothesis that the history of surgery—and to some extent the history of medical representation—is a history of touch as much as a product of visual practices and conventions.

The Artist and the Surgeon

Tonks decided to embark on a career in medicine at the age of sixteen, mainly, he later admitted, because it held more appeal than his father's other vocational suggestion, which was architecture.[7] With this goal in mind he became a student first at the Royal Sussex County Hospital in Brighton, and then at the London Hospital, where, in 1886, he was appointed house surgeon under Frederick Treves (the same year that Treves's best-known patient, Joseph Merrick, the "elephant man," moved into lodgings at the hospital, where he spent the last four years of his short life). In 1888, Tonks successfully passed his final examinations and became a fellow of the Royal College of Surgeons; more decisively, as it turned out, he also enrolled in evening classes at the Westminster School of Art with Fred Brown, who opened the door to the New English Art Club and eventually got him a job at the Slade School of Fine Art teaching drawing and anatomy.

Tonks was fifty-two when war broke out and an assistant professor at the Slade. By January 1915 he was working in a British Red Cross Hospital for the French in Haute-Marne, and was later posted at a clearing station nearby. He wrote to Geoffrey Blackwell: "The wounds are horrible, and I for one will be against wars in the future, you have no right to ask men to endure such suffering. It would not matter if the wounds did well but they are practically all septic."[8] Tonks realized very quickly that his medical skills were inadequate to the task at hand. "I have decided that I am not any use as a doctor," he wrote in another letter, after returning to London. "I don't think the Government very clever at using people's services. Munitions, anything in fact, I am ready to take up."[9]

Despite these misgivings, in January 1916 Tonks received a temporary commission as a lieutenant in the Royal Army Medical Corps. As well as assisting with operations at the new Cambridge Military Hospital at Aldershot, he had the unenviable job of assessing whether patients were fit to return to active duty. It was at Aldershot that Tonks met the pioneering plastic surgeon Harold Gillies. An ambitious New Zealander twenty years Tonks's junior, Gillies had convinced the authorities of the urgent need for specialist centers to treat the facial casualties arriving back from the front; he was appointed head surgeon at Aldershot when the center opened in 1916. It was Gillies who sought Tonks out, having heard from his friend (the *Times*' golf correspondent, Bernard Darwin) that "the great Henry Tonks" had been posted to Aldershot to work in the orderly room. In Gillies's biography there is a description of Tonks in his junior officer's uniform, looking much like "the Duke of Wellington reduced to subaltern's rank."[10]

A keen amateur artist himself, Gillies had taken drawing lessons by correspondence so that he could record his surgical procedures, and he recognized the value—both personal and professional—of working with such a talented draftsman. He asked Tonks to draw the patients before and after surgery, in addition to producing diagrams of the operations (Gillies continued to make quick sketches for his surgical assistants).[11] In April, Tonks wrote to his friend, the writer and art critic D. S. MacColl:

> I am doing a number of pastel heads of wounded soldiers who had had their faces knocked about. A very good surgeon called Gillies who

> is also nearly a champion golf player is undertaking what is known as the plastic surgery necessary. It is a chamber of horrors, but I am quite content to draw them as it is excellent practice.[12]

What can Tonks's fortuitous collaboration with Gillies tell us about the relationship between art and surgery, both in the context of wartime Britain and in relation to the broader histories of medical representation and aesthetics? These are not easy questions to answer: our protagonists were practical men, not writers or public intellectuals. We have little choice but to rely on anecdotal and circumstantial evidence, to take an oblique approach to questions of influence and motivation. In this chapter I draw two broad conclusions: that the nature of the injuries witnessed by Tonks and Gillies contributed to a heightened awareness (certainly on Gillies's part) of the *aesthetic* dimension of reconstructive surgery. Second, that Tonks's surgical training and experience made him highly attuned to the physicality, the *fleshliness* of art.

A Strange New Art

According to Gillies's biographer Reginald Pound, most general surgeons were embarrassed by facial wounds. The usual practice was simply to "pull the edges of the wound together, insert stitches and hope that nature would do the rest."[13] Gillies was determined to change all that. In France, he observed the renowned plastic surgeon Hippolyte Morestin and Charles Auguste Valadier, a dental specialist; he also studied photographs of the techniques used by German plastic surgeons.[14] "Appearance," he concluded of the German approach, "was of secondary importance." Indeed, "To a German the uglier the scar the more honourable the wound."[15] Even the French (who might be thought more "sensitive" to appearances) had neglected the aesthetic side of plastic surgery.[16] Gillies's biography turns on this pointed observation: modern plastic surgery—the unplanned child of modern medicine and modern war—was, above all, a "strange new art."[17]

For Gillies, the re-creation of a patient's looks—his human appearance—was as crucial as restoring physical function. He describes the procession of casualties returning from the western front following the Somme offensive of July 1, 1916. Two hundred extra beds had been set aside at Aldershot for facial casualties. Two thousand patients arrived. "Men without half their faces; men burned and maimed to the condition of animals."[18] As we saw in chapter 2, doctors and nurses were not alone in perceiving these injuries as dehumanizing. The tabloid press horrified and fascinated readers with descriptions of men "with their faces shattered beyond human semblance."[19] In a profound sense, appearance *is* function because one must be recognized as human to be treated with humanity.

Like the "strange new art" of facial reconstruction, Tonks's drawings blur the line between art and medicine; and by disturbing the conventional categories of medical illustration and portraiture, they highlight the ambiguities that lie at the heart of those representational practices. Approached as portraits, the drawings imply frankness and trust: one finds a suggestion of psychological depth and intimacy that is absent from the photographs of the same patients filed with the case notes.[20] Reflecting on the lessons he learned as a resident medical student, Tonks wrote:

> The medical profession stands alone in giving an observer occasion for a profound study of human beings, whether from the point of view of their structure, or—and this is even more interesting and perhaps important for the physician—the working of their minds. Everyone whatever is to be his calling in after life, would be the wiser for watching at the bedside of the sick, because the sick man returns to what he was without the trappings he has picked up on his way.[21]

For all their poignancy, Tonks's drawings, no less than the case photographs, are the product of specific institutions and conventions: medical and military, in the first instance, but also aesthetic and epistemological. The images and accounts of facial injury that have survived bear witness to physical and psychological trauma, but they also violently disrupt the cultural ideal of embodied masculine subjectivity. They are personal, empirical, *and* symbolic in equal measure. The complexities become apparent if one compares Tonks's pastel studies with other, more usual, forms of medical representation: graphic illustration and photography.

The Gillies Archives, now housed at the Royal College of Surgeons of England in Lincoln's Inn Fields, contain a wealth of visual material: pen-and-ink diagrams and X-rays as well as pre-and postoperative photographs, some in stereograph. The archives' former curator at Queen Mary's Hospital painstakingly matched the subjects of Tonks's portraits to the medical case files, making it possible to compare the pastels with photographs and other archival material (figures 45 to 49). The

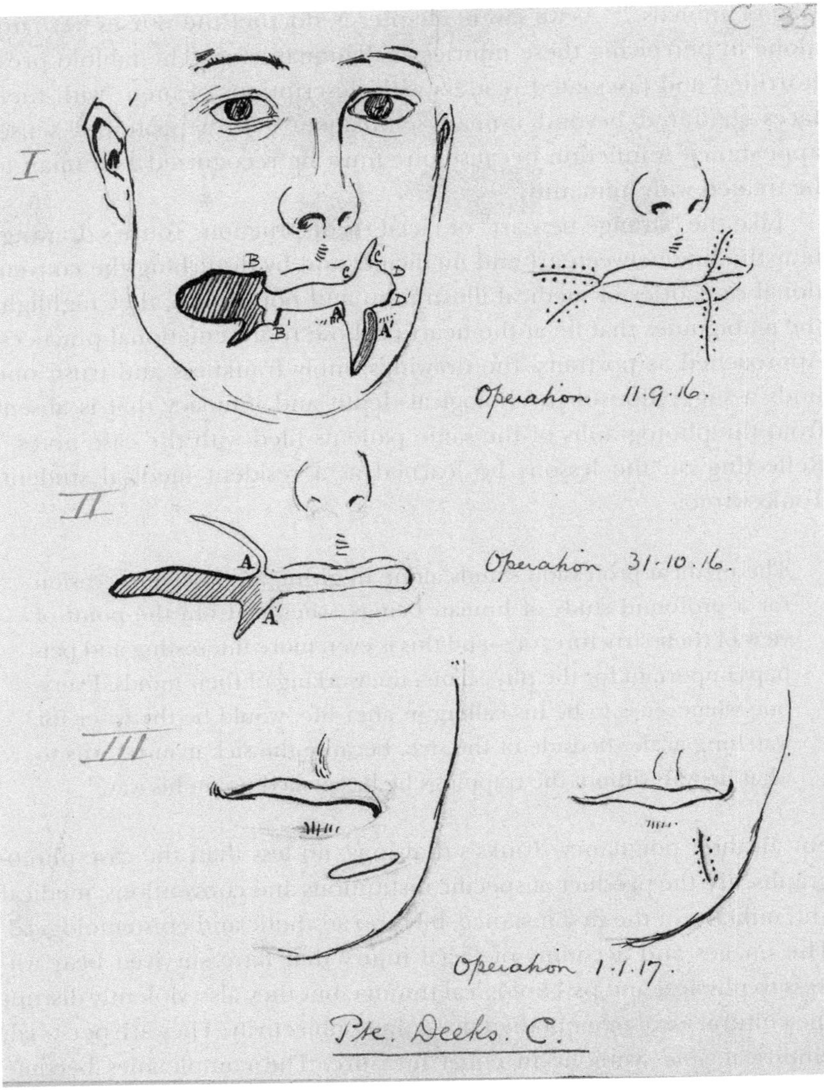

Fig. 45: Diagram by Henry Tonks from the Deeks case file from MS0513/1/1/ID553. From the Archives of the Royal College of Surgeons of England.

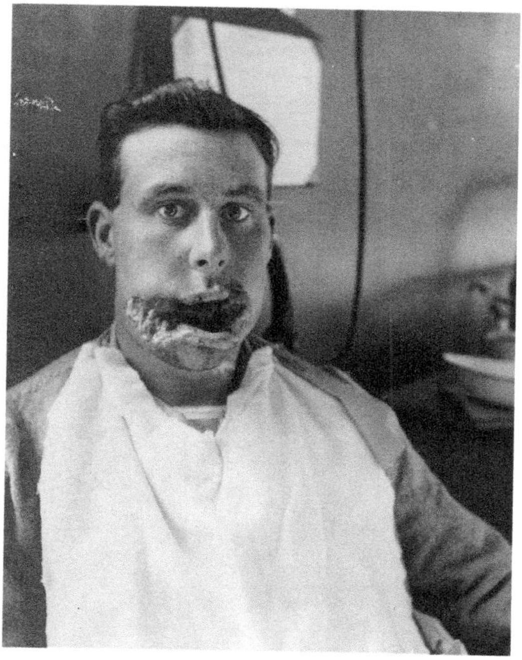

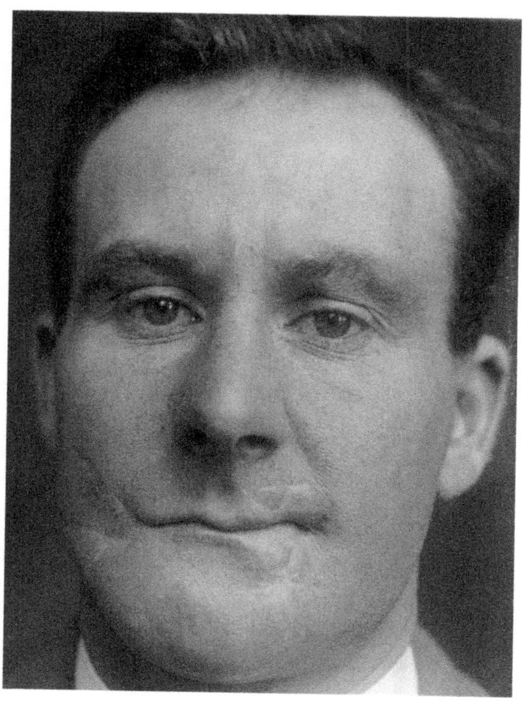

Figs. 46 and 47: Photographs from the Deeks case file of the patient before and after surgery from MS0513/1/1/ID 553. From the Archives of the Royal College of Surgeons of England.

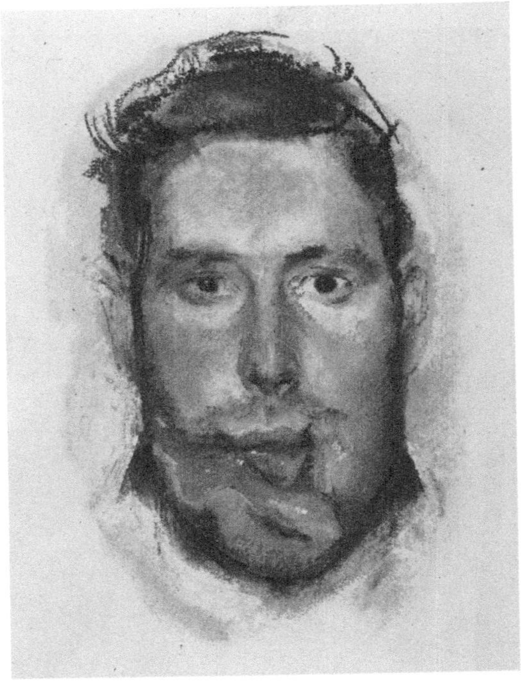

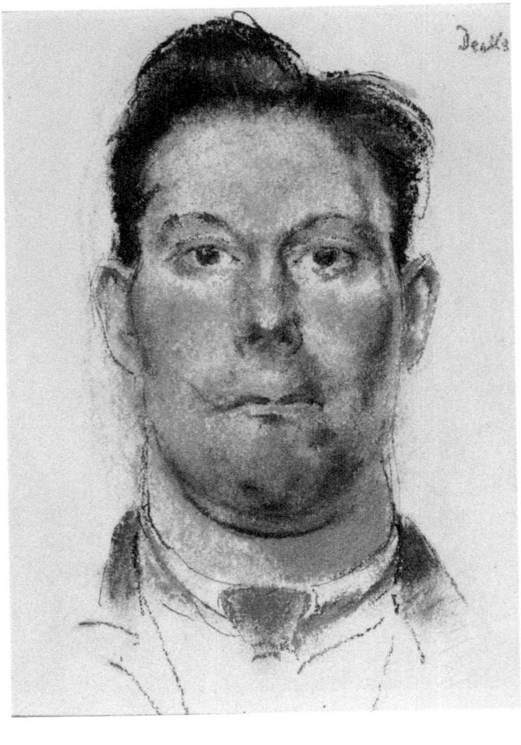

Figs. 48 and 49: Portrait of Private Charles Deeks, by Henry Tonks, 1916 and 1917, pastel. RCSSC/P 569.1 and RCSSC/P 569.2. (© Hunterian Museum at the Royal College of Surgeons.)

diagrams record Gillies's surgical procedures in the clearest and most economical form possible. Tonks has abstracted the wound from its human context, certainly from any suggestion of pain or suffering: there is not a hint of interiority, psychological or physical, apart from the jagged hollow of the wound. They have more in common with dress patterns than portraits, and indeed their purpose was instructive as well as documentary. To borrow a turn of phrase from the Royal Academy's first professor of anatomy, the obstetrician and surgeon William Hunter (1718–1783), the surgical diagrams are possessed of "a kind of necessary Inhumanity."[22]

Private Charles Deeks was twenty-five when he was caught in an explosion in France in July 1916 that obliterated much of his right cheek and mouth. His case notes include details of the wound, and the three operations to reconstruct his mouth. (Deeks was discharged to duty in April 1917 but survived the war, returning in 1919 and 1922 to have dentures fitted.) A preoperative photograph shows the extent of the damage (figure 46). Deeks would have been wearing a steel "Brodie" helmet—they were introduced in 1915—but although this increased his chances of survival, it did nothing to protect his face from shrapnel and flying shell fragments. Innovations in weapons technology were also responsible for new kinds of wounds that were larger and more complex than those inflicted by ordinary rifles.[23] The difficulty of producing "live" surgical diagrams in these circumstances is summed up by another artist who was posted to Sidcup and mentored by Tonks, the Australian Daryl Lindsay (1889–1976). Recalling his first operation, Lindsay reflected: "How was I going to translate what looked like a mess of flesh and blood into a diagram that a student could understand?"[24]

Medical drawing had always involved processes of selection and translation, as Chris Amirault explains: "To perform its medical work, only those details important to diagnosis [or surgery] should be emphasized, and other extraneous details should not."[25] The inclusion of incidental details—contextual, corporeal, aesthetic—presented a particular difficulty for nineteenth-century medical photography. This is what makes early medical photographs so fascinating as historical and cultural artifacts: unlike graphic illustrations, they inadvertently reveal *too much.* In the example we have just looked at, Deeks's upper lip forms a horizon beneath which his gaping lower face—the true subject of the photograph—is echoed in the crumpled neckline of a hospital gown. Above, we see the regular features and carefully combed hair of a good-looking young man.

Through the Camera's Eye

The artistic potential of photography was still being energetically debated in the opening decades of the twentieth century, but its empirical value had long been settled. Erin O'Connor notes that by 1859—just two decades after the invention of photography—photographs were being used to document disease in Germany, England, France, and America.[26] "Everyone agreed," she writes, "that the camera was an ideal scientific tool, far better than an artist's hand at recording the exact look of cells, stars, botanical specimens and human subjects."[27] But even the most objective-looking photographs rely upon series of technical and aesthetic manipulations: time is suspended; three-dimensional objects are compressed into two-dimensional shapes; living color (in the case of early photography) is converted to shade; and the subject comes into view through cropping and framing. We are struck by the incontestable evidence of "things as they are," but this conviction, writes O'Connor, has less to do with the camera's "accuracy," in the case of medical photography, than with its "capacity to conflate surface and substance, to present visual clarity as the key to the deep truth of disease."[28]

And yet photographs of combat injuries—like the one of Private Deeks—make no attempt to represent the invisible. What we see is all surface; or perhaps more correctly, the psychological depths alluded to in such photographs are uncharted.[29] In this respect, the medical photographs in the Gillies Archives are not equivalent to nineteenth-century studies of hysteria or photographs of the criminally insane (the images that have received most attention from historians of photography), which presented a legible body, an expressive surface—no matter that the meanings attributed to these bodies were little more than fantasies.[30] Even pictures of disease, and diagnostic medicine itself, relied on a visual semiotics linking visible signs to a "deep" pathology that was invisible to the naked eye. O'Connor develops this point, noting that advances in microbiology from the mid-nineteenth century contributed to a radical reconceptualization of disease. The study of cells revealed that disease was not a *thing* as such, in an ontological sense, but "the result of local or systemic deviations from normal physiological functions."[31] By contrast, wounds and surgical techniques clearly do have tangible, ontological existence. Surgery is a supremely material specialism.

The curiously entwined histories of nineteenth-century medicine and photography have been the subject of considerable scholarly interest, and it is not my aim here to add to this literature.[32] Rather than appealing to an overarching or underpinning history of medical representation—in which the medium itself is the continuous thread—I want to emphasize the social, institutional, and aesthetic contexts in which a particular group of images, photographs and drawings, were made and seen.[33] This necessarily involves some differentiation at the level of spectatorship: not all viewers are the same, and the meanings of images are a product of their framing—physical and conceptual—as much as their content and media. As a drawing instructor, Tonks was more aware than most of the extent to which we *learn* to see.

Many historians of photography—certainly those writing about its legal, military, and scientific (or pseudoscientific) uses—have been less interested in these nuances of spectatorship and context than in the role of photography as an apparatus of documentation, surveillance, or control. Our understanding of Victorian photography in particular is "distinctly Foucauldian," O'Connor remarks: "Photography was the agent of an oppressive objectivity, the argument goes; under cover of pure mechanical mimesis, it projected a distinctly political visuality."[34] Power, in this version of the modern disciplinary society, is anonymous and ubiquitous. Like the inmates of Bentham's panopticon, we never know when we are being observed or by whom, and so assume continuous surveillance. Lisa Cartwright's *Screening the Body: Tracing Medicine's Visual Culture* exemplifies this approach to the "medical gaze"—not a way of seeing so much as an impersonal, panoptic visuality; the product of new visual technologies (from the microscope to motion pictures) and new bodies of knowledge (in this case, modern physiology). It is, by her own admission, a book that "can perhaps be faulted for taking to an extreme the thesis that the cinema was used in science as a strategy of control and domination."[35]

While the political investments and social effects of medicine—and photography—must not be underestimated, these concerns are not directly addressed here. What I share with the broader poststructuralist project is something more subterranean: a wish to excavate the idea of representational "truth" in its historical setting. The relationship between truth and representation is a perennial topic in art history and visual culture, but in the context of war it acquires a heightened urgency. On March 6, 1914—some four months before the assassination of Archduke Franz Ferdinand in Sarajevo—Lord Haldane, the Lord Chancellor, gave the annual Creighton lecture at University College London on "The Meaning of Truth in History."[36] To an audience that included the Italian, German, Austrian, Russian, Japanese, and Spanish ambassadors, the provost and vice-chancellor of the university, and a host of MPs and judges, he posed this question: What should be the historian's "standard of truth?"

"The historian," he answers, "surely must resemble the portrait painter rather than the photographer." Like any great artist, the true historian possesses the ability to fathom the spirit of an age; to "disentangle the significance of the whole from its details and to reproduce it." His basic methods should be scientific and impartial, but ultimately, "art alone could . . . make the idea of the whole 'shine' forth in the particulars in which it was immanent." This ability to elucidate and breathe life, or the illusion of life, into the past distinguished the historian from the chronicler or biographer who amasses facts rather than interpreting them, a distinction made rather vividly by Sir Edward Grey in his opening remarks of the evening:

> A mere accumulation of facts and records could as little, without interpretation, give a true impression of the life, the spirit, the work, and the thought of a past age as a drawer full of dried and unmounted skins could give an impression of the life of birds in the air, on the earth, or on the water.

Few people today would be persuaded by this portrait of the oracular historian, finding in the dusty detritus of past events an essential, luminous truth. The convictions expressed by Sir Grey and Lord Haldane are very much of their time, but they do shed light on the equivocal status of photography during the 1914–18 war, and the comparative privileges enjoyed by the war artists.[37] The empirical status of the photograph as evidence relied on an appearance of unmediated reality; the belief that nature had represented *itself* without human intervention (aesthetic or ideological). This "reality effect," as Roland Barthes would much later describe it, lent the documentary photograph—and the photographer—a kind of innocence: a point that Sue Malvern makes in relation to World War I photography. Regarded as "craftsmen providing a service," the official war photographers had less authority, commanded less respect, and got paid less than artists like Paul Nash, Wyndham Lewis, C. R. W. Nevinson, or indeed Henry Tonks.[38] Paintings and photographs of the war were often compared, and the comparison usually centered on the question of truth: the camera's indiscriminate eye contrasted to the artist's ability to select and interpret, to invest a scene with *emotional* veracity. Jan Gordon's review of an exhibition of Canadian photographs at the Grafton Galleries in 1916 underlines this perceived difference between the artist and the camera (the photographer's presence is, as often, elided). Contrasting a photograph of a trench littered with German corpses with Nevinson's *La Patrie* of the same year, Gordon concludes: "'This is war,' cries the camera, 'as I see it.' 'This is war,' says Mr Nevinson, 'as I understand it.' And herein lies the difference."[39]

The Pastels

Tonks's studies of plastic surgery patients have not received much commentary, but a handful of essays have been published in addition to, and largely dependent on, Joseph Hone's discussion in his biography of the artist.[40] The most striking discrepancy in this small body of writing concerns the question of clinical or artistic objectivity. Hone claims that "Tonks brought a spirit, now of scientific, now of artistic detachment, to his task,"[41] a view endorsed in J. P. Bennett's supplement for the *Journal of Plastic Surgery*.[42] For Bennett, "One only has to see for a moment the Tonks pastels to be struck by the mastery of technique which records traumatized tissues; scarring, edema, salivary fistulae."[43] Gillies credits his colleague with the "foundation of the graphic method of recording [surgical] cases."[44] The Tonks who emerges from these accounts is, in Hone's assessment, "the historian of facial war injuries":[45] precise, accurate, detached, but also humane. Bennett insists that the drawings are more powerful than photographs "because the artist has, in a sense, instilled his sympathy and understanding into the record."[46] Julian Freeman is equally convinced of the superiority of Tonks's chosen medium over photography: "In each pastel, skin tones, mass, shape and color all appear, all of them beyond the reach of the camera."[47] Again, the drawings are described as "both accurate and impressive in their clarity."[48] Aside from the formulaic comparison with photography (to which we shall return), what interests me is the possibility of seeing the drawings differently: as unclear rather than exact, exploratory rather than definitive.[49]

Tom Lubbock finds in Tonks's pastels an aesthetics of ambiguity that is distinctively, if unintentionally, modern. This is not, however, the modernist distortion or abstraction of the figural found in, say, Picasso, Otto Dix, or Francis Bacon. The deformations of cubism and expressionism are, he points out, consistent, but Tonks's faces are affecting precisely because they are *violations* of formal and symbolic logic. They combine the familiar and the alien. The injuries are read, or rather they are unreadable, because we encounter them in the context of a perfectly ordinary face, with tousled or combed hair, details of clothing: the collar of a dressing gown, the knot of a tie; an engagingly direct gaze. In the midst of all this reassuring normality the ambiguously rendered injuries are "signal anomalies."[50] Emma Chambers makes a similar observation about the viewer's response alternating between "a horrified gaze at the areas of wounded flesh, and an attempt to locate the inner identity and personality of the sitter through reading emotions (of pain, resignation or bravery for instance) into the eyes."[51] This "mismatch" between "bodily presence" and "identity" is both disturbing and compelling: it sets in motion a compulsive, self-conscious gaze: exactly the kind of immoderate visual engagement that Tonks disapproved of. He clearly felt his own fascination to be superior to that of "all the more tedious visitors" to the hospital for whom the studies, framed and displayed in the artist's office, were one of the unmissable "sights."[52]

Is it possible that the wounds, in Tonks's studies, are ambiguous but also perfectly accurate and clear? Might my perception of undifferentiated flesh (or "bodily presence") be different from that of an expert: someone with detailed anatomical knowledge or surgical training? Lubbock is aware of this possibility, and quotes Tonks's admission that he had "often wondered . . . what the figure looks like to anyone who has not this knowledge [of anatomy]."[53] At the London Hospital, Tonks had the job of conducting anatomy demonstrations for students; in his autobiographical "Note from 'Wander-Years'" he recalls "bribing the *post mortem* porter . . . to fix a corpse on the table for my benefit, which I could then draw at my ease." His drawing skills were honed in the dissecting room and on the hospital wards: "Each patient," Tonks writes, "had a double interest, that of the disease which brought him there, and his possibilities as a model and how I would express them."[54] Tonks and Gillies would have been able to fill in any visual gaps with their own knowledge of the tissues and structure of the face, a form of knowledge that was tactile and instrumental as well as visual. One person's suggestive ambiguity is another's clinical detail, and to try to judge which is the more correct interpretation is to miss the point that accuracy and precision are partly in the eye (and fingers, and memory) of the beholder. There is no anonymous viewer on whom to pin our theories of spectatorship, and even the "medical gaze" is too blunt an instrument to account for the particular skills and sensibilities of a surgeon, a radiographer, an obstetrician.

Pastel is an accommodating medium. Because it requires no preparation or drying time between layers (like oils), it lends itself to improvisation and, unlike watercolor or pen and ink, a pastel sketch can be reworked. It is, on the other hand, a medium completely unsuited to archival documentation. Sticks of dry pigment mixed with a nongreasy binder, pastels are essentially pastes of colored dust—a form to which they all too easily return if not handled carefully. In his definitive *Grammaire des arts du dessin* (1867), Charles Blanc described pastel as an "exquisite powder":

> The lustrous and tender flesh-tints, the down of the skin, the bloom of a fruit, the velvet of fabric, cannot be better rendered than with these crayons of a thousand nuances which can be vigorously juxtaposed or melted with the little finger, and whose impasto seizes the light. Their soft, blond aspect, strengthened by some decisive browns, ravishingly expresses not only the brilliant tint of a young girl, the flesh of an infant, the finesse of a hand, the glisten and transparency of skin, but also certain delicacies of colour that oil mixtures might ruin.[55]

Pastel had long been associated with the feminine in art; a point that Anthea Callen makes in her study of Degas: not only was it popular with women artists; the medium itself was described in feminine terms.[56] It was used primarily for the "lowest" subjects in the academic hierarchy: still life, landscape, portraiture. Tonks was very much part of this tradition, and would have been familiar with the conventional distinction—invoked by Blanc—between line and color. "By implication," writes Callen, "pastel colour was soft, feminine, frivolous; oil colour was strong, vigorous, manly."[57] There is no frivolity in Tonks's Aldershot and Sidcup studies, but his choice and treatment of the medium emphasizes the youthfulness, fragility, and beauty of his sitters, as well as suggesting the fleshliness of their injuries.[58] It also gives the drawings a tenderness that is wholly absent from the photographs (and from Daryl Lindsay's watercolor portraits of the same men, which were painted from photographs). While the photographs record the horrific nature of the injuries for posterity, the pastels seem more fleeting, more time bound. They participate in their subjects' vulnerability and mortality rather than documenting it.[59]

Saline Infusion (figure 50) shows how masterfully Tonks could exploit these effects. Drawn in 1915 at the Red Cross hospital in Arc-en-Barrois, the religious overtones are hard to miss: this is, as Chambers suggests, a contemporary pietà or deposition:[60] the cross now a metal bed; the

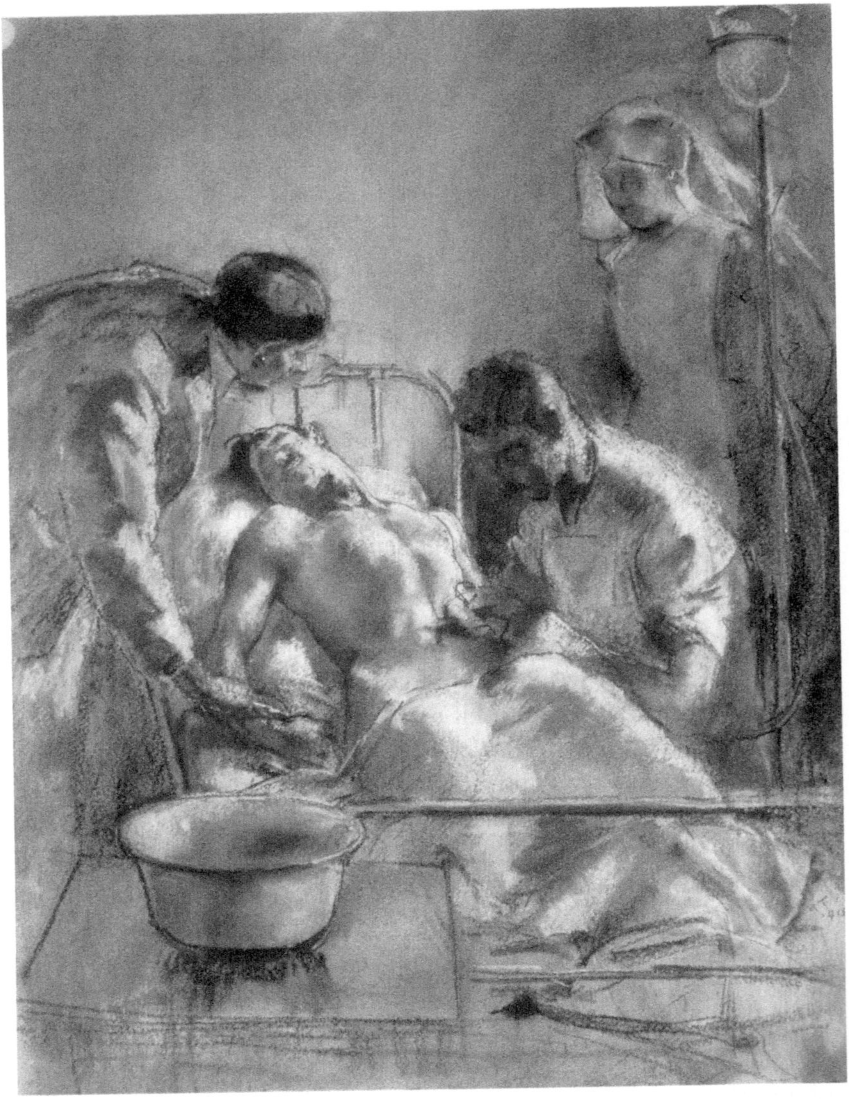

Fig. 50. Henry Tonks, *Saline Infusion: An Incident in the British Red Cross Hospital Arc-en-Barrois*, 1915, pastel, 67.9 × 52 cm. (Reproduced by permission of the Trustees of the Imperial War Museum, London.)

instruments of the Passion replaced by instruments of salvation, the needle and line of the saline drip highlighted in the same red chalk that outlines the wounded soldier's naked torso and neck. Exhibited the same year, the central figure was described by Sir Claude Phillips as a "magnificent young Hercules," a "splendid nude torso,"[61] yet—like many depictions of the crucified Christ—the hero is offered up to the viewer as thoroughly enfleshed object of desire. The tension between his Herculean appeal and his eroticized vulnerability has everything to do with Tonks's handling of his materials and the contrast between line and color, chalk and pastel. Callen remarks on the "direct physicality" of pastel in Degas's hands; the way he leaves raw marks unblended, creating lines that describe the female form but retain an independence from it. Like Degas's pastel drawings, Tonks's portraits are "palpably tactile but, of course, physically untouchable: they encode the sensation of touch—both the artist's touch and the experience of touching skin."[62]

We will come back to this question of tactility, but there is one further point of reference for Tonks's drawings to consider first. As we have seen, the surgical studies do not quite fit existing models of medical representation, graphic or photographic. The same can be said of traditional portraiture. Joanna Woodall observes that naturalistic portraiture has always been motivated by the desire to "overcome separation,"[63] to make the absent present, to reconcile image and identity, to defy death. None of this is possible without an experience of recognition. Yet in Tonks's drawings of wounded soldiers, the subject is doubly alienated from himself. In the first place, the institutionalization of these men (first in the military, then as long-term and usually recurrent residential patients) dislocates them from the social and physical fabric of their ordinary lives, their sense of a past and future meaningfully connected to the present. As well, the privileged signifier of subjectivity, the face, now signifies trauma. To a surgeon the damaged tissue may be a challenging text to read, but ultimately legible; to a pioneer in facial reconstruction the absence of a face may signify its potential surgical and prosthetic reconstruction, but to most of us, including perhaps the subjects themselves, the injuries are an abyss. The men Tonks encountered were capable of stoicism, even cheerfulness: one young man is described as "modest and contented" despite having had "a large part of his mouth . . . blown away,"[64] but these remarks are as disorienting as the remnants of traditional portraiture: the residual fragments of individuality conveyed through posture, gaze, clothing, and framing, fragments that only foreground the devastating violence of the injury.

These are antiportraits, in the sense that they stage the fragility and mutability of subjectivity rather than "*consolidating* the self portrayed."[65] Tonks himself referred to them as "fragments" in a letter to MacColl.[66] The achievements they celebrate are not those of the men we see (though to be alive at all was an achievement of sorts). The personality, the hero, of these untitled portraits is the pioneering surgeon, his inventiveness, skill, and dedication told through the simple narrative structure of "before" and "after." There is, however, another dimension to the drawings, another way of reading them against the grain of both conventional portraiture and medical illustration. Tonks's notion of verisimilitude, of visual truth, rested less on the certainties of anatomy than on a commitment to drawing as *practice.* Thomas Monnington offers some insight into the meaning of "practice" at the Slade. Drawing was understood as a process of research, "a really exhaustive search," he explained in an interview with Andrew Brighton.[67] "At the Slade there has always been a degree of experimentation—an unfinished quality. They painted pictures at the [Royal] College and they painted experiments more at the Slade."[68]

Drawing by Touch

Approached as iconic likenesses, the drawings unsettle the pictorial conventions and ideology of portraiture. The intrusion of the flesh disrupts traditional notions of subjectivity.[69] But seen as *drawings,* as marks on paper, the studies have an indexical rather than iconic quality: they no longer signify a person (hero, victim) or idea (the horrors of war, medical progress); instead, they present a material transcription of a sustained visual-tactile encounter. There are traces of earlier marks, evidence of reworking and layering. "All works of art are a series of corrections," Tonks wrote to his former student Rodney Burn in 1932.[70] The studies are densely worked but unfinished: some areas have a vigorous, linear clarity, while elsewhere, layering and blending creates a skin-like softness and opacity. One is drawn in by all these textural details: saliva glistening on the surface of a lip, the sharp tip of an ear or smooth parting of hair, a blush or smudge of pigment. None of this is adequately conveyed in reproductions. The drawings are completely different in the flesh; the compelling details of surface texture are lost in photographic translation, along with the sense of intimacy created by the scale (roughly half life-size) and material proximity of the drawings and the evident delicacy and duration of the artist's touch. In the originals, the wounds aren't revolting, the taut sheen of scarred skin is not grotesque. There is something at once exquisite and inhuman about the underface as Tonks depicts it. Tonks was proud of them, confessing to his former student Dickie Orpen not long before he died that they were the only drawings he was "not ashamed of."[71] They are personal, verging on private; not just because of the physical and psychological exposure involved, but because of the intimate visual-tactile encounter that remains implicit, indeed embedded, in the work.

Tonks wrote virtually nothing about his philosophy of drawing, did not give formal lectures, and generally disliked the art-theoretical discourse propounded by "art boys."[72] Apart from a report on the teaching of drawing prepared, with Sir George Clausen, for the Girls' Public Day School Trust, and passing references in Tonks's letters, we have to rely on the writings and reminiscences of his students. A set of maxims formed the backbone of his instruction: that drawing is very difficult; that practice is everything; that learning to draw is learning to see (and the inability to draw is an inability to see); that "literary" concerns (such as narrative or symbolism) have no place in pure drawing; that drawing is at its most truthful and affecting when it is directly observed, unidealized, and selfless.[73] The authority of these values flows from the French realist tradition defined by Courbet and Millet in the 1840s and 1850s, although Degas and Manet were more immediate influences.[74] From the very beginning, the curriculum at the Slade was informed by the French system of art education, with its elevation of the living model over study from the antique.[75] When the Slade School of Fine Art opened its doors to students in October 1871, it was under the professorship of Edward Poynter. Poynter, who came to the Slade from the Parisian atelier of Charles Gleyre, pledged to instill in his students "the knowledge of their craft at their fingers' ends before they began to paint pictures"—an implicit criticism of the competition.[76] In his view, students trained in the English system were all too often motivated by commercial gain rather than artistic mastery. Poynter was succeeded as Slade Professor by Alphonse Legros, then Frederick Brown, and, in 1918, Henry Tonks.

The most systematic account of the Slade philosophy of drawing is an essay by Tonks's student John Fothergill, who edited an official illustrated volume, *The Slade*, published in 1907.[77] In "The Principles of Teaching Drawing at the Slade," Fothergill introduces a paradox that animates Tonks's portraits of wounded soldiers a decade later: drawing (or in this account, great drawing) is fundamentally tactile. Touch is for the draftsman what sound is for the musician: a student who draws "by sight" is no better off than a deaf man who learns to play the piano by mimicking the movements of his instructor.

A good drawing, for Tonks, was one that conveyed a palpable sensation of the object—an "idea of touch"—whether a waxy apple or the curve of a model's back. "There are drawings," remarks Fothergill, "which make us feel that the draughtsman has been learning at every touch."[78] They have nothing to do with precise measurement or proportion, the abstract perfection of a line, an accurate contour, or a recognizable silhouette. The beginner is advised to think of the model as a "corporeous unity; hold this, and the line and shading will follow without you or your critic's being conscious of it."[79] "Corporeity" is not quite what it sounds. Rather than being an attribute of objects (their "materiality" or "fleshliness"), "corporeity" is defined in a footnote as the sum of an individual's visual-tactile experiences: the "result of our having from infancy unconsciously observed the light and shade on, and peculiar to, every form we have touched or traversed."[80] So when you describe an artist's "delicate touch," "rough handling," or "nervous feeling," these phrases are to be taken quite literally because "They tell us the manner in which the artist visually touches or handles form."[81]

The history of surgery, too, is partly a history of touch: technologically extended and transformed by the invention and refinement of surgical instruments. In art and in surgery, touch (or hapticity, the visual approximation of touch) can be diagnostic, interrogative, analytical, instrumental, or creative. Gillies describes how the initial examination of facial wounds could take up to a week, and involved manual palpitation to determine the extent and type of tissue lost (skin, soft tissue, bony substructure). The operation was planned with the aid of a sculptural model of the face, showing the missing contours, and radiographs to reveal any displaced bone or other material. The eventual operations demanded "the greatest delicacy of touch."[82] The visual appearance of injuries could be misleading: one patient's "enormous gaping wound," caused by an explosion, healed well with only minor surgery. Gillies's point is well illustrated by the before and after photographs in *Plastic Surgery of the Face*. The camera, he cautions, "occasionally represents an inaccurate conception of the wound."[83]

In Fothergill's essay, the "exactitude of the photograph" is analogous to the drawing done purely by sight. The mechanical representation of nature, whether by means of a camera or with the aid of measuring devices and techniques, *reveals* nothing. It has "merely duplicated the aspect of the model, minus the colour, and the spectator is no better off than he was before he saw the drawing. It has told him nothing. Being conceived with no ideas of tangible form, it gives him none."[84] Tonks despised the "snapshot" approach to drawing,[85] but his hostility toward photography is also consistent with his disparaging view of scientific (specifically industrial and technological) "progress," mechanization, and mass production (of which cubism was, in his view, symptomatic). Not surprisingly, his subjects were, with the notable exception of the wartime studies, untouched by modernity: family scenes, sunlit interiors, the occasional landscape, ladies' portraits, everything gently and charmingly familiar. There is a preponderance of female subjects in Tonks's work: "The paintings," notes Stephen Chaplin, "are often of young women yearning after contemporary critics knew not what,"[86] and it is tempting to see this affinity with the domestic and the feminine as an aesthetic retreat from the historical present. For Chaplin, Tonks's best-known work is "poised between the eighteenth and nineteenth centuries."[87]

Toward the end of his life Tonks urged Rodney Burn (then the director of the School of the Museum of Fine Arts in Boston) to read Gina Lombroso's *The Tragedies of Progress* for an account of the "bad 20th century": "It is a remarkable explanation of views I have held ever since I read Ruskin nearly 50 years ago."[88] Tonks's opinion chimes with a deep vein of pessimism, in English and Continental European thought, about the social and cultural effects of industrialization and mechanization; a deep suspicion, too, about visuality in a world seemingly dominated by the mass-produced spectacles (photographic and cinematic) of the popular media and entertainment industry. But Tonks was no cynic where art was concerned. Hone notes that a brand of Schopenhauer-inspired mysticism was very much "in the air" and can be detected in Tonks's conviction that art, far from being a "mere embellishment of life," was "the one really worthwhile, the redeeming, activity of mankind."[89]

Tonks did not always make a pleasant impression on his students, many of whom—including Paul Nash, Richard Nevinson, and Percy Wyndham Lewis—went on to redefine British modernism as they attempted to represent the Great War.[90] It is easy to see the differences between teacher and students as evidence of an unbridgeable generational divide, and to agree with Nevinson that art must spring from the same source as war—the same currents of violence and mechanization—if it is to truly give form to the experience of modern combat.[91] But in *The Modernity of English Art*, David Peters Corbett reminds us that modernity is not "dependent on modernism for its realisation in the cultural sphere."[92] We should, writes Corbett, be more attentive to different "*types* of relationship—explicit, withdrawn, evasive, direct—to the experience of modernity."[93] Lisa Tickner's *Modern Life and Modern Subjects* is an example of what can be achieved by "expanding the frame" to encompass "a cultural history of representations of modernity, rather than an art history of canonical modernists."[94] In Tonks's case, as in many others, the artistic response to modernity was deeply (and irreconcilably) contradictory. Tonks was by no means alone in his nostalgic attachment to an imaginary world untouched by modernity, but he was also fully engaged with a corporeal present that was inescapably modern because formed (and deformed) in the crucible of modern, mechanized combat.

The comment is often made that Tonks's knowledge of anatomy stood him in good stead as an artist and drawing instructor. Reading Fothergill's essay suggests rather different priorities, to do with the embodied knowledge and manual, tactile experience acquired through surgical training and practice in the dissecting room. At the same time, Tonks interrogates the idea of beauty (and by extension, that of ugliness or the grotesque). Through dedication and practice, one might, he believed, achieve "a kind of intimacy," but "only by seeing the thing itself . . . from painting the thing." To his friend Mary Hutchinson he admitted that such intimacy was not always pleasant: it might lead "us into the most squalid places, almost holding one's nose."[95] Helen Lessore recalls being taught by Tonks in the 1920s:

> In his preaching of "Truth to Nature" Tonks managed to convey a moral quality, a conviction that Beauty was somehow incidental, a side product of the pursuit of Truth; that it would be a reward unexpectedly discovered in the most unpromising material, provided that we followed certain disciplines and were faithful to our experience.[96]

For me, there is a productive tension in Tonks's World War I pastels between the sensuous appeal of his medium and the shock of seeing the seriously injured body. In this they recall Degas's drawings of prostitutes whose striated flesh bore traces of the artist's lingering eye and hand. Far from the virginal ideal of untouched and untouchable femininity, Degas's bathers seemed to be marked by "marriages, childbirths and illnesses," and contemporary audiences reacted with disgust as well as fascination.[97] As with Tonks's drawings, the ambiguity of Degas's figures is easy to miss in reproduction: what the critic Gustave Geffroy described as a "distressing poem of the flesh" in 1886 has become a popular subject for poster art.[98] This is not likely to be the fate of Tonks's studies, but in both cases "beauty" is redefined as an intense aesthetic encounter rather than as a visible quality of beautiful objects.

Tonks was aware that every artwork has its own life; that the drawings he was so satisfied with could be "dreadful" in a different context. Unapologetically elitist, he produced drawings at Aldershot and Sidcup with two kinds of viewers in mind—medical and artistic—both, in his view, professional. And yet, as I have suggested, the drawings themselves are troubling even *within* these contexts precisely because they blur the line between them. I have described them as antiportraits, but they have an equally complicated relationship to medical representation because their intimacy and incidental beauty undermine the "necessary inhumanity" of clinical medicine.

CHAPTER 5

The Afterlife of Henry Lumley

In 1997 the Hayward Gallery in London put on a touring exhibition called *The Quick and the Dead: Artists and Anatomy*. In the book accompanying the exhibition Ludmilla Jordanova reflected on the points of contact and dissonance between these two pursuits, art and anatomy: a history encapsulated in the title of her essay, "Happy Marriages and Dangerous Liaisons." The study and representation of the human body has, since the Renaissance, been constrained by practical and moral considerations—a limited supply of cadavers, the politics of patronage, codes of decorum governing the circumstances in which a naked or dead body could be seen or depicted—but it is only in the last forty or so years that artists have openly exploited the subversive potential of medical themes and images. "Indeed," writes Jordanova, "in recent decades, medicine has supplied the materials with which artists can openly explore the troubling, unsettling aspects of bodily phenomena."[1]

This chapter concerns one such troubling liaison between medicine and art, although computer games are not often described as art, or have not been until very recently.[2] Jordanova mentions the "huge impact of photography in making widely available a disturbing literalism": literalism being one of the attributes most often associated with "dangerous" images.[3] Game designers are equally invested in the production of reality effects through computer graphics and sound. In the case explored here, the use of medical records as source material was intended to enhance the game's realism, and therefore its potential to frighten (or "unsettle" to use the term preferred by contemporary critics). But there is another reason to begin a discussion of medical archives and digital culture with Jordanova's remarks on artists and anatomists. One of the achievements of the Hayward exhibition was to dislodge the idea of historical context as something singular (as in "it must be seen in context") and to suggest, instead, the multiplicity of contexts and audiences. "For each image," Jordanova reminds us, "there are innumerable contexts, since they are constantly being transplanted and transformed, re-viewed by each generation."[4]

Exhibiting Damaged Bodies

Some of the most powerful images of World War I—though not war art in the usual sense—are those in which art and medicine converge, as they do in Henry Tonks's delicate pastel portraits of British servicemen with severe facial injuries and the equally exquisite (and unsettling) prosthetic masks made by the sculptor Francis Derwent Wood for some of these patients to conceal their disfigurement when surgical reconstruction was impossible. In both of these examples, art could be said to ameliorate the horrors of war, and to humanize men who had suffered what were considered at the time to be the most dehumanizing of injuries. They are, to use Jordanova's expression, examples of the happy marriage of art and medical science: collaborations defined by mutual regard and a common goal. In both cases, however, the sources that have survived contain assumptions about how, where, and by whom the injured body may be seen—assumptions that have changed over time. This chapter considers the afterlives of some of these sources. When we encounter medical images in a museum or art gallery, or on a website like *Morbid Anatomy*, what kind of cultural and imaginative work do they perform?[5] Are there ethical considerations raised by their redeployment or appropriation within the contexts of art and entertainment, education and academic research?

I started thinking about these questions when I discovered that case photographs from World War I medical archives had been used in *BioShock*, a computer game designed by Ken Levine and released in August 2007. It won the BAFTA for Best Game that year, among a constellation of other awards, and is ranked in the top five Xbox 360 and PlayStation 3 games to date.[6] Over four million copies of the game have been sold. *BioShock II* was released in February 2010, and Universal Studios has plans for a film.[7] Without giving the plot away, this is a spectacularly gory game, and some of the most memorable encounters are with genetic mutants known as splicers. It is these subhuman monstrosities that bear an uncanny likeness to Tonks's portraits and the case photographs of the same men housed in the Gillies Archives at Queen Mary's Hospital in Sidcup.

Tonks, as we've seen, regarded his surgical studies as inappropriate for public consumption, and complained of the visitors to the hospital who treated the drawings as one of the "sights." In recent years though, the portraits have found a wider audience. They have been exhibited at the Venice Biennale, Tate Britain, London's Science Museum, the Hunterian Museum at the Royal College of Surgeons of England, Wellcome Collection, University College London, and the National Army Museum in Chelsea. In June 2007 the full series was made digitally available on the website of the Gillies Archives,[8] and Pat Barker has spoken of them as an inspiration for her novel *Toby's Room*.[9] The photographs of Gillies's patients have entered the public domain alongside the drawings. A selection of complete case files from the Gillies Archives was put online as part of the Wellcome-funded sci-art collaboration Project Façade, and case photographs have featured in several recent exhibitions including *Faces of Battle* at the National Army Museum and *War and Medicine* at the Wellcome.[10] Even more than the drawings, the photographs question the limits and propriety of spectatorship. At least with the pastels, one is aware—almost physically—of Tonks's attentiveness, the quality of the artist's touch, and the duration of his gaze. His authority, as an artist and surgeon, licenses our own interest. The photographs appear unmediated by any aesthetic concerns: physically and psychologically naked.

Cocurated by the artist Paddy Hartley and the NAM's education officer, Samatha Doty, *Faces of Battle* presented extensive documentation of facial injury in World War I Britain alongside textile sculptures. Working in collaboration with Andrew Bamji at the Gillies Archives, and with the help of a genealogist, Hartley used photographs, texts, and oral history to piece together the stories and experiences of some of the men whose faces were rebuilt by Gillies and his team. These images and narratives were incorporated into digitally printed and embroidered military uniforms and facial "garments" (as Hartley refers to them), each ensemble a composite portrait of one man. Dwelling as it did on the devastating brutality of modern combat—and the political and social burden of sacrifice—I expected the exhibition to be controversial. It opened in November 2007, at a time when dead and wounded

British soldiers were off limits to embedded photojournalists in Iraq and Afghanistan; yet here were British casualties of war, on public display, in an institution not otherwise known for drawing attention to the human cost of armed conflict.

Flipping through the visitors' book on a quiet Friday morning in summer 2008, it was clear that people had found *Faces of Battle* harrowing, disturbing, gory, upsetting, or—in the words of one young visitor—"gross & it made me feel sick."[11] But they had also been deeply affected, describing the exhibits as amazing, humbling, and "cruel but real."[12] "This has been the most moving exhibition related to any war that I have ever seen," wrote one visitor; "thank you for bringing home to the public the human pain of war so often lost in museums."[13] Most of those who left comments made no mention of Hartley's interpretive pieces. What they seemed to value was the immediacy and "reality" of the objects on display, the photographic records, letters and case notes, surgical instruments, and plaster casts of disfigured faces: a reality inseparable from (or perhaps guaranteed by) their shadowy half-life in medical archives.

The exhibition's subtitle was "Untold Stories of Suffering, Heroism and Hope," and although there was plenty of undiluted horror on offer, the curators did their best to convey a positive message. Like HBO's *Alive Day Memories*, *Faces of Battle* was framed by an ideology of heroic sacrifice and medical progress. "Advances in medicine and surgery have often come as a result of developments in weapons and technology," one text panel explained, echoing the words of Sir Clifford Allbutt (and a great many other surgeons and historians of medicine): "How fertile the blood of warriors in raising good surgeons!"[14] In an entry on war and medicine in the *Companion Encyclopedia of the History of Medicine*, Roger Cooter unpicks the logic of "progress through bloodshed" that underpins these narratives of sacrifice and hope.[15] He points out that medicine never develops purely in response to the medical needs of individuals. In times of war, medical progress is driven by a paradoxical ideology: "Its primary goal is not to preserve health for the sake of individuals, but for the for sake of destroying the might of others. . . . [F]rom the combatant's perspective, war is not good for medicine so much as medicine is good for war."[16] The American surgeon Fred Albee makes a similar point in his memoirs:

> Perhaps it is as well that a surgeon in a military hospital is too overworked to have time to think. To use all the skill and ingenuity you possess to heal a shattered body so that it may be useful again to stop

more bullets, does not bear thinking of. And in the military hospitals of France there was no time for thought.[17]

A broken soldier is a useless weapon, and the ultimate purpose of the army medical corps was to return men to active service.[18] Military medical archives embody this paradox—which turns the preservation of life into the potential for death—and this, perhaps, is one of the reasons why medical images of mutilated soldiers are usually so well guarded.

When I teach this material (usually to history of art and museum studies students), I tend not to use the most harrowing images of facial injury and reconstructive surgery. Apart from my own mild squeamishness, I worry how my students will respond: with pity, disgust, or fascination? Should I name the patient, I wonder, or protect his anonymity? Would he, or his relatives, want the photograph to be shown in a nonmedical context? Is there a happy ending—a redemptive "after surgery" to counterbalance the "before"? These questions might give me pause for thought, but they generally remain unspoken. Here, though, I have chosen one image precisely because it confronts the interested, curious, or appalled viewer with the problematic nature of spectatorship and empathy. The photograph in question (figure 52) is a preoperative record of one of Gillies's patients, who was also drawn by Tonks: Henry Ralph Lumley. Figure 51 shows Lumley before his injury. These photographs, like the other images reproduced in this chapter, can be found quite easily on the Web, along with Lumley's case notes, a series of photographs documenting the operations, and Tonks's portrait.[19] When I last checked, the preoperative photograph had more than 250,000 hits, so either it has been seen by a considerable number of individuals, or there are people—like me—who've returned to it repeatedly, for whatever reason.

Henry Lumley was admitted to the specialist hospital for facial casualties in October 1917. In his notes, Harold Gillies describes Lumley's condition on admission: the skin and subcutaneous tissue of his face had been destroyed by severe petrol burns, including the left eye and eyelid, both eyebrows, and the nose down to the cartilage. A second lieutenant in the Royal Flying Corps, Lumley had been wounded on July 14, 1916: By the time he came to Sidcup, he had lived with his injuries for over a year. No further mention is made of the accident in the case notes, but a genealogist working on Project Façade looked up Lumley's service records in the National Archives.[20] A former operator with the Eastern Telegraph Company, Lumley was selected for the RFC's Special Reserve

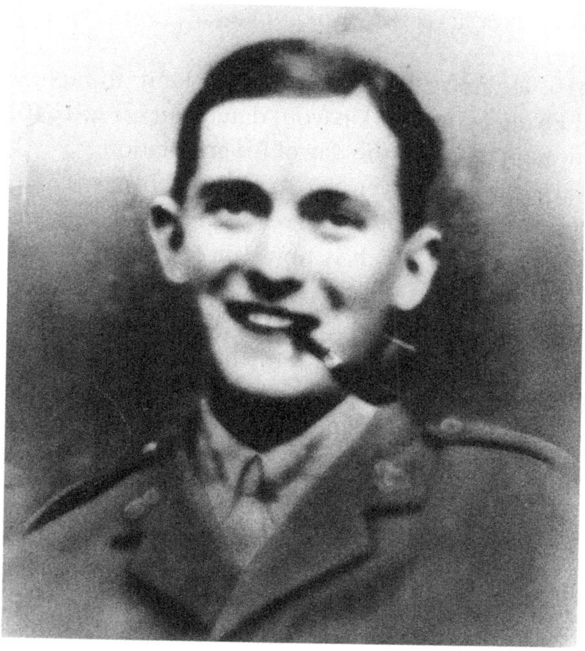

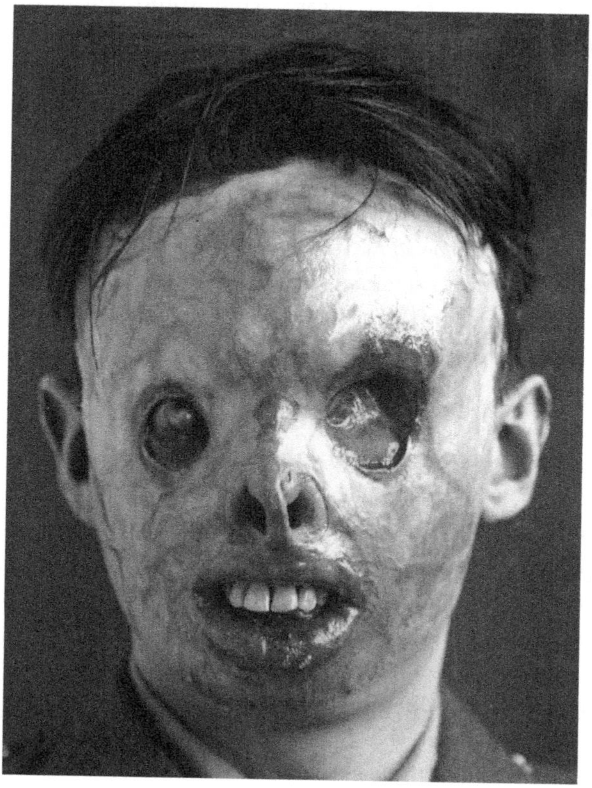

Figs. 51 and 52. Pre and postinjury image of the patient, from the Lumley case file from MS0513/1/1/ID 1284. From the Archives of the Royal College of Surgeons of England.

of Officers in April 1916. He never made it out of England, though: a letter from the Central Flying School in Upavon, dated August 9, 1916, reveals that the accident happened on the day of his graduation.

The two operations at Sidcup, in November 1917 and February 1918, are documented in detail in the case notes, and revisited in Gillies's 1920 textbook, *Plastic Surgery of the Face,* which is now out of copyright and freely available online.[21] A diagram (figure 53) shows Gillies's ambitious plan to remove the existing scar tissue and raise a large flap of skin from Lumley's chest, with pedicle tubes providing a further blood supply to the graft. Despite ongoing complications, the initial signs were encouraging, but by day 3 after the second operation the graft had developed gangrene. Henry Lumley died twenty-four days later on March 11, 1918. He was twenty-six.

The Burdens of Representation

What do we gain from seeing images like these? What would constitute their proper—or improper—use? Susan Sontag's book *Regarding the Pain of Others* (2003) is probably the most famous attempt to answer this question. In it she returns to the scene of her earlier essay, *On Photography,* and reconsiders the claim, almost three decades on, that we (in the West) have become desensitized to the suffering of others; that this moral anesthesia is directly attributable to the proliferation of images of appalling suffering. In *On Photography* Sontag pointed out an innate paradox of photographs: that they could, simultaneously, make an event *more real* than if one had never seen the photograph, but also—through "repeated exposure"—*less* real.[22]

Regarding the Pain of Others is not easy to précis. Despite its urgency and brevity it is a book in which conclusions proliferate. Here are just a few of Sontag's arguments, each one a serviceable truism:

> No "we" should be taken for granted when the subject is looking at other people's pain.[23]
>
> Being a spectator of calamities taking place in another country is a quintessential modern experience.[24]
>
> The problem is not that people remember through photographs, but that they remember only the photographs.[25]
>
> Harrowing photographs do not inevitably lose their power to shock. But they are not much help if the task is to understand.[26]
>
> Our sympathy proclaims our innocence as well as our impotence.[27]

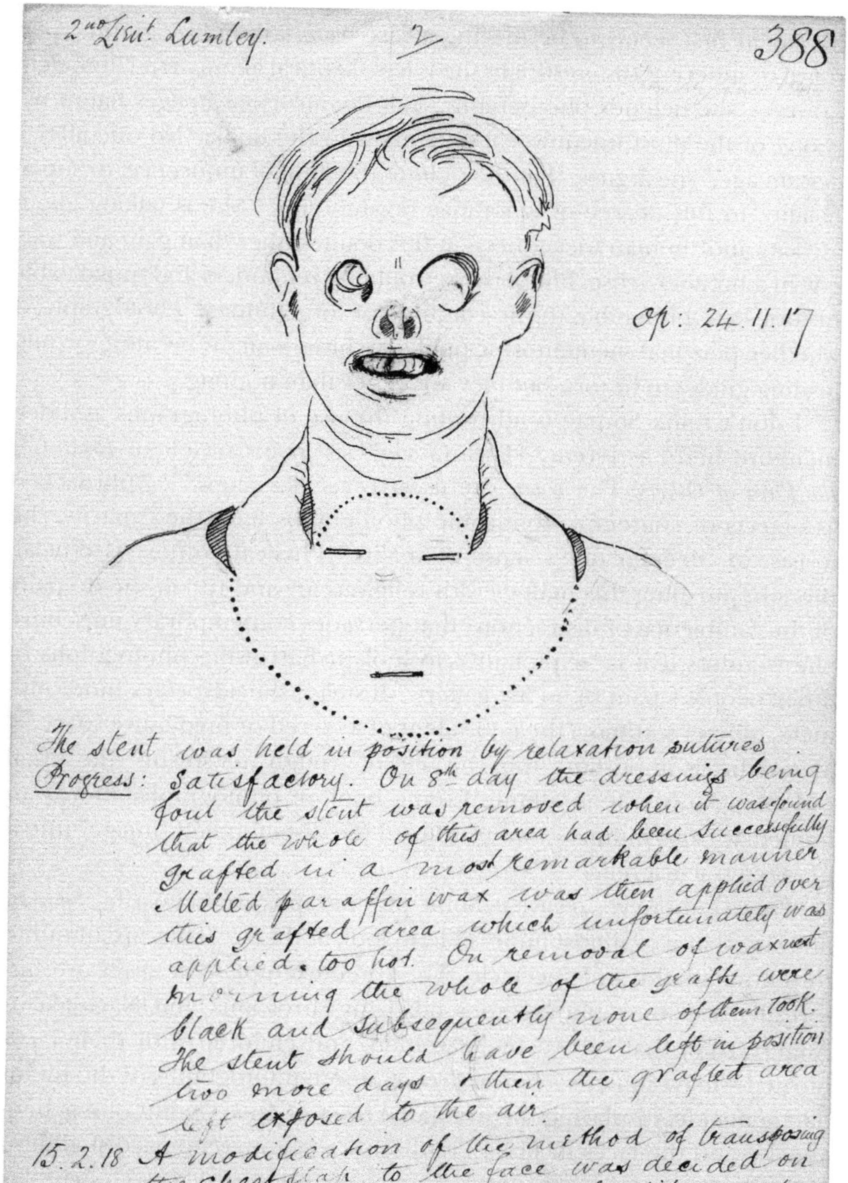

2nd Visit Lumley. 2 388

Op: 24.11.17

The stent was held in position by relaxation sutures
Progress: Satisfactory. On 8th day the dressings being foul the stent was removed when it was found that the whole of this area had been successfully grafted in a most remarkable manner. Melted paraffin wax was then applied over this grafted area which unfortunately was applied too hot. On removal of wax next morning the whole of the grafts were black and subsequently none of them took. The stent should have been left in position two more days & then the grafted area left exposed to the air.
15.2.18 A modification of the method of transposing the chest flap to the face was decided on & one extra pedicle on each side was added to the scheme. Note photograph.
" " " General condition fair but there has been very little attempt at regeneration of the raw area from which the neck pedicles were

Fig. 53. Diagram by Henry Tonks from the Lumley case file from MS0513/1/1/ID 1284. From the Archives of the Royal College of Surgeons of England.

Sontag at first seems to be making a case *against* the photographic portrayal of suffering (interestingly, she is less skeptical about art). Ultimately, however, she defends photography. "Let the atrocious images haunt us" is one of the most unequivocal statements in the book: "No one after a certain age," she argues, "has the right to this kind of innocence, or superficiality, to this degree of ignorance or amnesia."[28] She is talking about atrocity and "human wickedness" at this point, rather than pain and tragedy in a broader sense, but perhaps troubling reminders and unpalatable histories are preferable to the comforts of forgetfulness. Photographs—whether personal mementos or public archives—might be mute or misleading guides to history, but they are better than nothing.

I don't think Sontag is advocating the use of photographs as aides-mémoire here, as Jeremy Harding suggests in his review of *Regarding the Pain of Others*. The term she uses is "secular icons."[29] Approached as objects of contemplation, some photographs have the capacity, she insists, to "deepen one's sense of reality." Physical context is crucial, though: pursuing the analogy with religious art and ritual, she despairs of the "ambience of distraction" that pervades contemporary museums. She wonders if it is "exploitative to look at harrowing photographs of other people's pain in an art gallery." Instead, she advocates more intimate, quieter settings, "the equivalent of a sacred or meditative space."[30] Materiality is important, too: the feel of "rough newsprint," the ritual of looking through an album. Even a book of photographs affords an immediacy and intimacy that transform the disembodied "image" into a material trace: a relic.

There is, however, a caveat. Some photographs are so horrific, Sontag reasons, that it is almost impossible to look at them.[31] They are immune to sentimentality and spectacle. The three examples she gives are historically disparate: photographs taken in Hiroshima and Nagasaki in August 1945 that record men, women, and children with their faces burned—like Lumley's—beyond recognition; photographs of the Rwandan genocide, displaying the mutilated faces of Tutsi victims of machete attacks; and the faces in Ernst Friedrich's 1924 anarcho-pacifist album, *Krieg dem Kriege!* (*War against War!*).[32] In a chapter titled "Das Gesicht des Krieges" ("The Face of War"), Friedrich reproduced twenty-four photographs of German soldiers with facial injuries: the exact equivalent of the images in the Gillies archives. By confronting the public with these *Schreckensbilder*—horror pictures—he hoped to stem the rising tide of German militarism (hence "War against War"). There is, Sontag insists,

> shame as well as shock in looking at the close-up of a real horror. Perhaps the only people with the right to look at images of suffering of this extreme order are those who could do something to alleviate it—say the surgeons at the military hospital where the photograph was taken—or those who could learn from it. The rest of us are voyeurs, whether or not we mean to be.[33]

When the photographs of Lieutenant Lumley and Gillies's other patients were taken, they were certainly never intended for the curious or contemplative or horrified gaze of the general public: not because of patient confidentiality laws, which didn't exist, but because of the nature of the injuries, which were considered potentially demoralizing. The public response to facial disfigurement was then (and still is) characterized by aversion.[34] As we saw in chapter 2, aversion can take many forms, from the institutional and social isolation of "facial" patients and the efforts made to conceal disfiguring injuries, to the relative invisibility of disfigured servicemen in the wartime press and propaganda.

These acts of disavowal and erasure create a dilemma for historians, and for anyone dealing with the visual record of facial mutilation and disfigurement in the contexts of publication, exhibition, or education. The stigmatization of servicemen with facial injuries was, and is, clearly reprehensible; and there is a powerful case for making disfigurement and disability (and "difference" in general) much more visible. It is in this spirit that the British charity Changing Faces launched its Face Equality campaign in May 2008, challenging negative perceptions of facial disfigurement. One of their strategies is to encourage the media, film industry, and advertisers to "adopt more factual and unbiased portrayals of people with disfigurements."[35] One of the studies they cite—analyzing 8,650 hours of British television—recommends (among other things) "more people with disfigurement in front of and behind the camera."[36] We cannot, now, restore Gillies's patients to their place in society; but we might give them a place in history.

Yet representation—indeed visibility itself—can be a burden as well as a privilege. Writing in the 1980s, John Tagg detailed the "burden of subjection" implicit in legal, medical, and police photography in the last decades of the nineteenth century.[37] The wish *not* to be represented—not to be exposed, or made public, or held up as an example, or pitied, or studied—is surely something to be mindful of, particularly in cases like Lumley's, where there is no possibility of collaboration or consent.

Rapture

While I was looking online for images from the Gillies Archives, I came across a discussion forum hosted by 2K Games. 2K—formerly Irrational Games—is the developer of *BioShock*, a first-person shooter game critically acclaimed for its narrative complexity and artistic ambition. This is how the game's copywriters describe the story:

> After your plane crashes into icy uncharted waters, you discover a rusted bathysphere and descend into Rapture, a city hidden beneath the sea. Constructed as an idealistic society for a hand-picked group of scientists, artists and industrialists, the idealism is no more. Now the city is littered with corpses, wildly powerful guardians roam the corridors as little girls loot the dead, and genetically mutated citizens ambush you at every turn. BioShock forces you to question the lengths to which you will go and how much of your humanity you will sacrifice . . . to save your own life.

The online discussion is headed "Project Façade vs Bioshock?" and begins on July 18, 2007, amid the flurry of publicity just prior to the game's release.[38] The original posting is simply a set of links: the first takes you to Project Façade, the second to Henry Lumley's photograph, the third to one of the concept drawings for *BioShock* (figure 54), and the last two to stills from the game itself (figure 55).[39] The debate circles around a series of questions: Did the game's designers use real people (Lumley is not alone) as inspiration for the monstrous inhabitants of Rapture?[40] Does that matter? Will it change the way you play the game, knowing that the enemy you are shooting, bludgeoning, or blowing up is based on someone who was shot, burned, or blown up for real? Are there, in other words, ethical limits to artistic "inspiration," on the one hand, and immersiveness or realism on the other?

One has to bear in mind, of course, that this is a site for players who are probably going to buy and enjoy the game regardless. For them, *BioShock*'s "creepiness" and moral ambiguity are its greatest virtues. "This just excites me even more," posts "Poopypooperson" (the most dogged witness for the defense) at 11:51 on Wednesday night: "the level of detail they put into the game, that these portraits existed before! Should make it even scarier playing it in the dark at midnight because of all this historical depth to the design."[41] "I am freaked out indeed," adds "I love Mr Bunny" just after midnight, "but I don't get why people are saying that

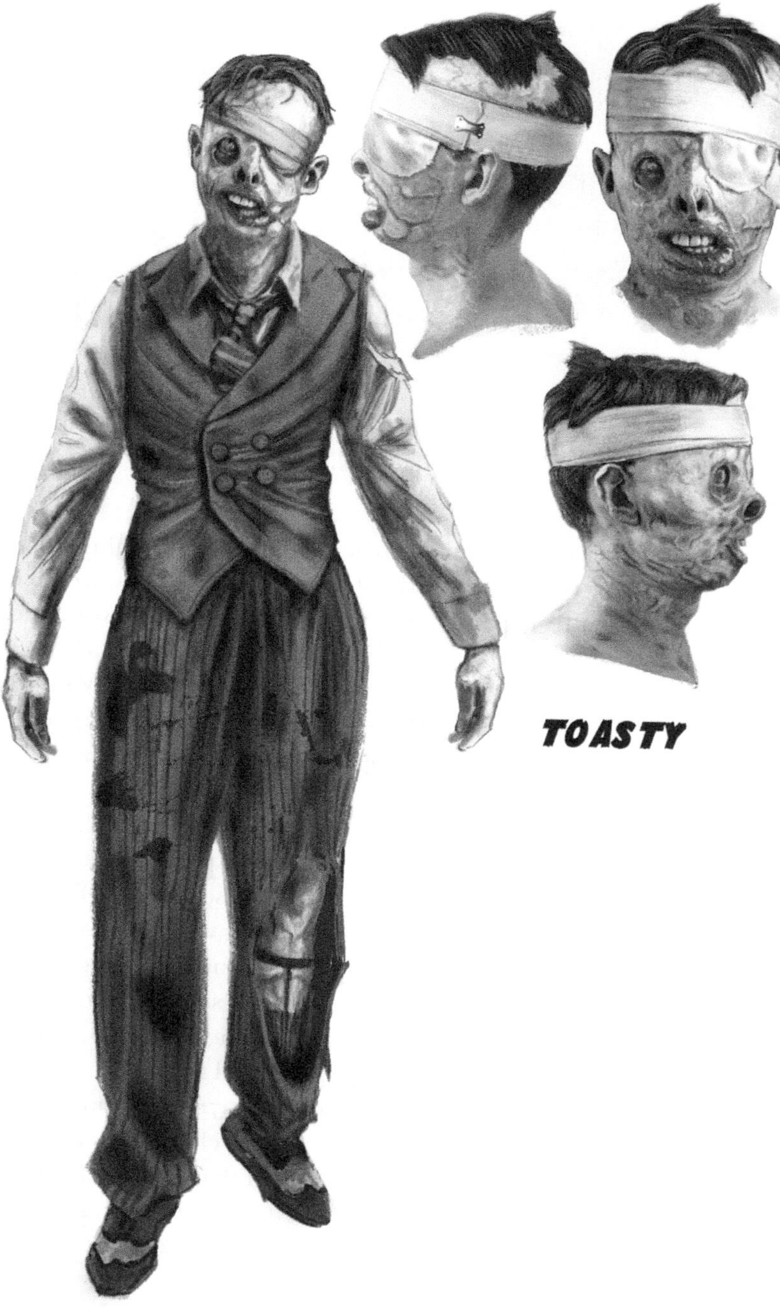

Fig. 54. Concept artwork for the "Toasty" model in *BioShock*. Take 2 Games.

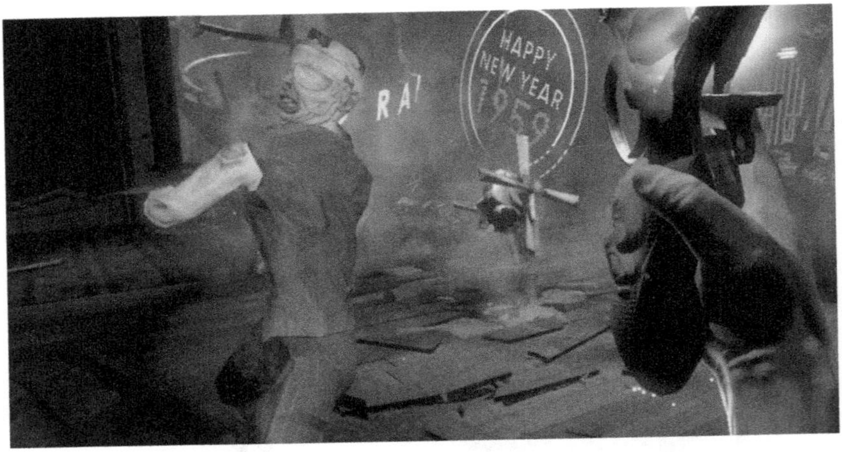

Fig. 55. *BioShock* screenshot. Take 2 Games.

it's bad to copy."[42] Picking up the thread on Thursday morning, "godot" points out that the concept artwork "was quite obviously inspired by the 90 year old images from Project Façade. But IG isn't sell [*sic*] concept art. They are selling a game in which the facial textures for a few characters were developed from concept art that was inspired by some 90 year old images."[43] "Well, it's clearly more than just 'inspiration,'" objects "CodeMonkey": "It looks like the artists traced his character's face directly from the original photograph."[44]

As the afternoon wears on, forum members mull over the legality of Irrational's use of the Project Façade material. "There had to have been some kind of contact between the two sources," reasons "Bioshock_FTW." "I think they'd know how much of a legal war they'd end up in over something as sensitive as this without asking permission first."[45] Godot reports that he "looked across that site and saw no indication anywhere of copyright notice. Most of the images come from an old hospital archive. If by chance they were ever copy protected then someone would have had to renew their copyrights in 1947, 1975 and 2003 to keep them falling into the public domain."[46] Then he changes tack: "Ok, all legalities aside for a moment . . . Did IGN label that concept art [of the character based on Lumley's photographs] TOASTY?" It's just a name, replies Poopypooperson. "Just a name, huh?" responds godot. "What if the concept art was based on a Holocaust victim and they named it 'RABI' [*sic*]'?" Poopypooperson's answer, posted on the Friday afternoon, is worth quoting in full:

> We aren't fighting WWI veterans in this game, we're fighting people that were surgically enhanced so [as] to survive in the harsh environment Rapture. The game's depression and horror qualities are masked by an extreme dark humor that further incites the insanity running rampant within Rapture's borders. Part of this dark humor is the spiteful nicknames given to these miserably derelict people, it's evocative of freak shows and human zoos, if you will. Of course it's cruel! Nobody should be mocked for features they can't control, are they going to be mocked though, without a question! Cruel, yes, but only because it's realistic based on human nature to discriminate [against] those who don't look like us.[47]

There have been several sustained attempts to think through the ethical implications of violent computer and video games, including a special issue of the *International Review of Information Ethics* devoted to "The Ethics of E-Games" (2005).[48] Variously informed by moral philosophy, computer game theory, literary and cultural studies, phenomenology, and social psychology, this nascent interdisciplinary field has several distinguishing features: a fairly unanimous desire to defend computer games and their players from tabloid stereotypes of mindless and addictive violence; and an understanding of ethics and morality as something *internal* to the game experience: the interaction between a designed object (with elements of narrative, game world, and game play) and a rational, creative, morally reflective subject (the player). Miguel Sicart's book *The Ethics of Computer Games* is the most recent contribution to this project. Taking his cue from virtue ethics (a theory first formulated by Aristotle), Sicart asks a simple question: does playing a particular computer game make you a good or bad person? Is it, in other words, a virtuous thing to do? He concludes that the player of a computer game is "a moral user capable of reflecting ethically about her presence in the game, and aware of how that experience configures her values both inside the game world and in relation to the world outside the game."[49]

It would be hard to disagree with Sicart that computer games "are now what cinema and rock and roll once were: the bull's-eye of morality."[50] *Why* this should be the case he doesn't say. An exercise in applied philosophy, *The Ethics of Computer Games* does not, unfortunately, pursue historical questions of cause and context. It is an approach that has its uses—not least in defusing moral panic—but it produces a peculiar blindness when it comes to the question of violence. In Sicart's vivid analysis of the game world, the "world outside the game" hardly exists at all. In a book on ethics this is problematic to say the least, because it fails to consider any possible interaction between fantasy and reality. The psychological effects of playing violent computer games—and their wider social ramifications—simply remain questions in need of "further development."[51]

BioShock is the perfect case study for Sicart because moral choices and consequences are built into the game, making it a kind of labyrinthine *Pilgrim's Progress.*[52] Rapture—a darkly sumptuous "City of Destruction"—is a testament to the corrupting power of human greed and untrammeled individualism. Built in 1946 as a utopian experiment, it is now (circa 1960 in the game) in a state of terminal but beautiful decay. *BioShock*'s lead designer, Joe McDonagh, explained in an interview that the developers wanted to

> create a game which deals with moral shades of grey and doesn't try and patronize us with two-dimensional cut outs. . . . We thought that gamers are mature enough, sophisticated enough to deal with sophisticated moral issues.[53]

The artists who worked on *BioShock* are surprisingly open about their sources.[54] In the *Making of BioShock* DVD, which has been posted on YouTube, Nate Wells (one of the technical artists) admits—slightly uncomfortably—that the Project Façade website provided "disturbing inspiration" for their splicer artwork.[55] Within the game, surgery serves as an allegory for the progressive commodification of the body/self in late capitalism.[56] Having passed through the first level of *BioShock,* Welcome to Rapture, players find themselves in the Medical Pavilion: a cross between a fairground house of horrors and an art deco theater.[57] Ornate double doors swing open to the sound of maniacal laughter, a bell chimes ominously, neon lights flicker on and off, and water pours through a crack in the ceiling. Posters advertising "Dr Steinman's Aesthetic Ideals" are taped haphazardly to a wall adjacent to the Funeral Services entrance. Another pair of doors leads into the operating theater itself. Through a wire grille we see the surgeon in what appears to be a soiled butcher's apron and scrubs. The source of the blood soon becomes apparent: Steinman is repeatedly stabbing his patient with a scalpel, oblivious to the fact that he now has an audience. This is not a place to linger: fleeing the surgery, we pass more posters marked BEFORE and AFTER. On closer inspection, the pretty woman in the "before" image has also suffered at Dr. Steinman's hands. In blood, on the wall below, someone (the mad doctor himself?) has written, "AESTHETICS ARE A MORAL IMPERATIVE."

BioShock does not pretend to be a facsimile of the social world—there isn't even any dialogue—but it does offer novelty, spectacle, showmanship, and good old-fashioned shocks. Aesthetically, it has much in common with the "cinema of attractions" of contemporary horror films.[58] In the absence of dialogue, the backstory and plot are conveyed through "audio diaries" that the citizens of Rapture have made as a final record of their hopes, memories, and (in most cases) their demise. The effect is something like a "macabre radio drama," says Matthew Weise.[59] We learn from listening to these diaries that the Medical Pavilion was built as a state-of-the-art general hospital for the citizens of Rapture. It all started to go wrong with the discovery of ADAM, a viscous substance harvested from parasitic sea slugs. When injected, the stem cells in ADAM caused genetic mutations in their human hosts that initially seemed beneficial. It soon became apparent, however, that excessive use of the drug had serious side effects. Users began to behave erratically and to exhibit strange physical mutations. Dr. Steinman—an enthusiastic user and advocate of the drug—experienced its psychological and physical ravages firsthand: a surgical mask only partially conceals his deformity when we meet him in the Surgery. Steinman's audio diaries record his descent into insanity: "I am beautiful, yes," we hear him muse in one recording. "Look at me, what could I do to make my features finer? With ADAM and my scalpel, I have been transformed. But is there not something better? What if now it is not my skill that fails me . . . but my imagination?"[60] In another diary he likens his genius to that of Picasso:

> When Picasso became bored of painting people, he started representing them as cubes and other abstract forms. The world called him a genius! I've spent my entire surgical career creating the same tired shapes, over and over again: the upturned nose, the cleft chin, the ample bosom. Wouldn't it be wonderful if I could do with a knife what that old Spaniard did with a brush?[61]

Splicers like "Toasty" show Steinman's ingenuity at its darkest.[62] Gillies's surgical experiments were groundbreaking and meticulously executed, but in the photographs they often look primitive: the postoperative faces of his patients like crudely stitched and unevenly padded doll heads. What is obvious, in *BioShock*, is that the idea—the *promise*—of plastic surgery has waxed and then waned over the past hundred years. The rhetoric of magical "repair" (and cosmetic "improvement") has lost its innocence. Biomedical technologies, genetic engineering, and the relentless marketing of health and beauty represent, for many, "a world from which humanity has been drained" rather than a world in which one has "unprecedented freedom to reinvent oneself."[63]

From horror films to hospital dramas, the contemporary medical imaginary is a place of fascination and dread. Above all, it is in the hospital—that "sanctuary of contemporary terror"—that the body's salvation and ruination is obsessively rehearsed.[64] As Pete Boss explains:

> Modern medicine, its methods of quantification and treatment, its technology and power, stands, at once, as that which improves or prolongs our (physical) existence, and the constant signifier of its limitations, a condition which allows it to slide rapidly from reassurance to disturbance in its imagery.[65]

Of course, artists since the Renaissance have used medical subjects and images for inspiration: from Leonardo da Vinci's grotesques to Francis Bacon's collection of medical textbooks.[66] When the contents of Bacon's studio in Reece Mews were posthumously cataloged by archaeologists, one of the items that came to light was a chromolithograph of diseased gums that Bacon had torn from a copy of the *Atlas-Manuel des maladies de la bouche*, a French translation of an 1894 German medical textbook, acquired while Bacon was in Paris in 1927 (figure 56). The scrap of paper shows "Fig. 1":

> a heavily retouched photo of lips prized apart by forceps to reveal gums disfigured by an abscess, chipped teeth, and froth about the tongue. The chromolithograph with its flesh reds stands as an oval vignette on the creamy fragment of coated paper. But then the scrap has been scuffed by brushes loaded with green and cerulean; there are fingerprints to the right in blue-black and mauve, little splats of yellow and scarlet.[67]

The gaping mouth of the *Atlas-Manuel* reappears throughout Bacon's oeuvre, most famously in the central canvas of *Three Studies for Figures at the Base of a Crucifixion* (1945) and the "screaming popes" of the 1950s. It cannot have crossed his mind to seek permission. What is the difference between Bacon's fascination with those "beautiful" diseased mouths—as

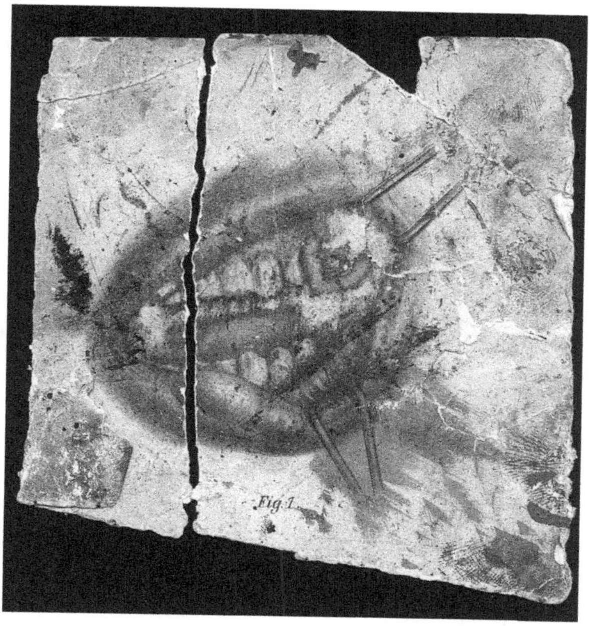

Fig. 56. Two fragments of leaf torn from the book *Atlas-Manuel des maladies de la bouche, du pharynx et des fosses nasales* by Ludwig Gruenwald, Paris: Bailliere et fils 1903. Hand-colored illustration depicting gum disease. From the Francis Bacon Studio. Collection: Dublin City Gallery The Hugh Lane. (© The Estate of Francis Bacon. All rights reserved, DACS 2014.)

he described them in a 1966 interview with David Sylvester—and the use of Gillies's case photographs in *BioShock*?

Is the difference that one is art, the other entertainment? Although the distinction is ultimately unsustainable, it is still widely believed that "art" is morally beneficial (except perhaps when it is too entertaining) and that computer games are not. In art (it is said) cruelty and violence are sublimated or contemplated rather than simply enjoyed. There is, however, a more tenable difference, to do with recognition and identity. To begin with, the mouths in the *Atlas-Manuel* are anonymous—unlike Gillies's patients. We recognize faces and names, and familiar voices, but not (unless you are a dentist or forensic pathologist) teeth or gums. Furthermore, the creative distance between the colored plate in the textbook and the eventual painting makes recognition impossible: even a dentist would fail to identify Bacon's sources from his operatic deformations of the human. The problem with *BioShock* is that the splicers are identifiable individuals, who—if they were alive—would be entitled to sue for defamation or slander. All of Gillies's patients are now dead, but many live on in the memories of their children and grandchildren. For them, *BioShock* can only be a perverse transgression of the pledge not to forget.

Reality Effects

Neither Project Façade nor the Gillies Archives were set up to deal with commercial clients or the finer points of copyright law. Curious how a larger organization might have responded, I contacted the head of Wellcome Images, Catherine Draycott.[68] The Wellcome has over forty thousand clinical and biomedical images in its online database, alongside over one hundred thousand photographs of paintings, prints, drawings, manuscripts, rare books, and archive material from the Wellcome Library collections. A search for historical images of plastic surgery turns up an album of World War I photographs from King George Military Hospital (later the Red Cross Hospital) in London: pictures that would have served the purposes of *BioShock*'s art department just as well as those featured in Project Façade.[69] Wellcome images are generally free of charge for study, teaching, and academic publication, but commercial use is chargeable and governed by specific terms and conditions.

The Wellcome's definition of "commercial" is wide-ranging, covering everything from the reproduction of images in medical textbooks to "artist reference" fees for CGI and special effects. If makeup artists on the BBC hospital drama *Casualty* need to make a gunshot wound look realistic, they can use photographs from the Wellcome Images database for reference.[70] Would the Wellcome have permitted the developers of *BioShock* to use their photographs in the game? No, said Draycott, they wouldn't: even though such a request might fall under the rubric of "artist reference," it would have been considered unethical. The comparison she made was Benetton asking for images for an advertising campaign. The problem was not the commercial use of medical images per se, but the fact that they were being used to shock. Even if the patient could not be identified, "The usage would still have been unethical."[71]

Leaving aside the unlikely possibility of a transatlantic copyright case, where does this leave Henry Lumley? Should we conclude that his ghostly presence in *BioShock* only "deepens the moral grey areas" of the game, to quote one forum member?[72] One of the problems with this conclusion is that it fails to address the concerns raised by players in the discussion forum, who point to a troubling interaction—or blurring—of real and imaginary worlds. In contrast to Sicart, who brackets the world outside the game, what disturbs the players (or some of them) is precisely the intrusion of the historical real. Here is the case against *BioShock*, from someone whose nom de plume is Nias Wolf:

> I just feel a little bad that we are using these poor souls (who fought in a war by the way) for entertainment. If I was disfigured horribly, and saw my face being portraid [*sic*] as a monster, I would be greatly offended.[73]

"I'd be surprised if they are still alive," replies I love Mr Bunny. "Well, they aren't, but they may still have families," points out Nias Wolf, adding a few posts later:

> Honor the dead people. And honor soldiers too. I just want to keep that in mind.[74]

One of the genuinely innovative—and truly eerie—things about *BioShock* is the way it incorporates found objects into the game world. One of these objects is Lumley's photograph, but the commitment to realism is not confined to the game's visuals. Each level or "deck" in Rapture has a different theme: the fisheries, the medical deck, Arcadia all have distinctive musical and ambient elements: aleatoric music, solo cello and violin, and jazz piano are interspersed with recordings of buoy bells and boats, the distant sound of a concertina, footsteps, a car horn, voices. "I actually found the sound of an insane woman on the Internet," Garry Schyman explained, "and messed with her voice digitally and infused it into the score, and it becomes a very scary element." Schyman, who composed the soundtrack for *BioShock*, cites musique concrète as an important influence on his score. He was asked to produce something "radically different . . . unique and experimental." The resulting montage of just under eighty minutes of orchestral music and incidental sound reflects his "very realistic approach."

In a lecture at the annual Game Developers Conference in 2007, Schyman gave his audience a sneak preview of the soundtrack. One of the clips featured what sounded like a man's dying breaths.[75] "I found a website of some doctor at a university," Schyman explained over the sound of labored breathing. "This is diseased breathing. I took his sick people breathing sounds and used it. I don't know if that's a copyright infringement." We will probably never know who the breathing man is, but his spectral presence in *BioShock* is as haunting as any of Sontag's photographs. Breath has ancient associations with the spirit or soul: our word "spirit" comes from the Latin *spiritus*, meaning "breath." The Greek term *pneuma* has the same double meaning. The pre-Socratic philosopher Heraclitus (535–475 BC), for example, believed that the afterworld was a place of smoky exhalations, where the souls of the dead intermingled.[76] The breathing in Schyman's score is a recording of a recording; just as Lumley's presence in the game is a computer animation of a drawing of a photograph, but there is something about these particular found objects that transcends the distance between the original and its representation. They perform what Roland Barthes called a "reality effect"—and in the process they bring us into uncanny proximity with the dead and the dying.

Allan Sekula referred to the photographic archive as a "'clearing house' of meaning,"[77] but in these cases the archive also seems an appropriate resting place, something perhaps best left undisturbed. Sekula, of course, was thinking of the photographic archive (as institution and aspiration) in its repressive nineteenth-century incarnations, as an apparatus of surveillance, classification, and social control. Photography, he argues in "The Body and the Archive," "came to establish and delimit the terrain of the *other*, to define both the *generalized look*—the typology—and the *contingent instance* of deviance and social pathology."[78] Medical photography is part of this history, but as I have argued in this book, it is far from monolithic in its aims or methods.

In a special issue of the journal *Photographies* titled "Photography, Archive and Memory," Karen Cross and Julia Peck note the persistence of Sekula's Foucauldian vision of photography. It has become difficult, they write in their editorial, "to conceive photography and the archive to involve anything other than the negative operations of power."[79] While acknowledging the necessity of the critique of photography pursued by Sekula and Tagg, among others, Cross and Peck set a new agenda: one that would begin with the excluded and the overlooked. A counterarchive, if you like, of residual or repressed images, memories, and meanings. It is a project, they suggest, that resonates with the "growing desire to salvage images produced in ordinary and everyday circumstances by ordinary people"—from the photos in family albums to the old black-and-white prints for sale at antique markets.[80]

On the surface there is nothing to connect our case study to either of these approaches to the photographic archive. The makers of *BioShock* are not interested in challenging the ideology or normalizing effects of medical archives: if they were aware of the Gillies Archives at all, it can only have been in the partial and highly mediated form of Project Façade. *BioShock*'s investment in historical veracity is entirely stylistic. As Frederic Jameson observed of nostalgia films and historical novels, what matters is conveying "pastness."[81] (The *BioShock* concept artist Robb Waters also mentions using "old mug shots from the 1940s.")[82] On the other hand, trawling the Internet for old medical and police photographs is not so different from rummaging through boxes of photographs at flea markets—or buying photographic memorabilia on eBay. If there is indeed a growing interest in (and market for) historical photographs, *BioShock* is part of the trend.

Context Collapse

The research for this chapter began with a personal question: I wanted to know why *I* was troubled by the ethics (as distinct from legality) of these acts of appropriation. From a historical or anthropological perspective, however, it is just as important to understand why some players in the forum are *not* worried about Henry Lumley's reincarnation in the game. For them, it seems, there is no imperative to contextualize, not in the sense that historians use the term. Indeed, the commonplace understanding of context—defined in the OED as "the circumstances relevant to something under consideration"—seems almost quaint when faced with the "circulations, reimaginings, magnifications, deletions, translations, revisionings and remakings" made possible by contemporary digital media.[83] The New York–based conceptual artist Seth Price has described the Internet as an "unruly archive" that lends itself to perpetual recycling. The artist's task, he writes in *Dispersion* (2002–),

> becomes one of packaging, producing, reframing, and distributing; a mode of production analogous not to the creation of material goods, but to the production of social contexts, using existing material. Anything on the internet is a fragment, provisional, pointing elsewhere. Nothing is finished.[84]

Price's understanding of context as something that is crafted serendipitously from found objects and images is very different from the idea of a preexisting substructure of determinate conditions (social, cultural, economic, environmental) that together generate and explain behavior and meaning. Ironically, the postmodern turn evident in Price's reflections brings us closer to the original use of "context" to refer quite literally to the joining together (*contextus*) of a book (from the Latin *contexere*, to weave together). One reason, then, why historical medical photographs might turn up in a video game is that they are perceived, in their digital form, as free-floating fragments; evanescent splinters of the past that exist in suspended animation, until an artist or blogger or game designer weaves them into a "context." As Price admits, this is necessarily a project that "encourages contamination, borrowing, stealing and horizontal blur."

The art-historical precedent for these strategies is, of course, the readymade,[85] but Price's comments invite comparison with a more recent cultural phenomenon: an experience that the anthropologist Michael Wesch terms "context collapse." Wesch is primarily interested in the ways in which new media like YouTube, Twitter, Facebook, and Flickr have altered people's perceptions of themselves and others. Since 2007, he and his students at Kansas State University have been charting the evolution of the video blog, or vlog. Uploaded onto YouTube at the rate of several hundred thousand per day, vlogs are often "deeply personal" and yet addressed to no one or dedicated simply to the "YouTube community."[86] For the first-time vlogger, faced with a recording webcam, the experience can be profound:

> The problem is not lack of context. It is context collapse: an infinite number of contexts collapsing upon one another into a single moment of recording. The images, actions, and words captured by the lens at any moment can be transported to anywhere on the planet and preserved (the performer must assume) for all time.[87]

Wesch is writing about the emergence of new forms of subjectivity and community, but "context collapse" offers a way of rethinking aspects of contemporary visual culture as well. It points to the heightened potential for what Price refers to as "horizontal blur": the loss of traditional boundaries and categories ("medical image," "documentary photography," "art," "entertainment"). This isn't always a bad thing, but it does coincide with an erosion or disavowal of other kinds of difference. Wesch tells the story of the *One World* video by MadV, which attracted a record two thousand responses when it was posted on YouTube in 2006.[88] The original forty-one-second video showed an anonymous hand reaching toward the camera, the words "ONE WORLD" written on the palm in black marker pen. Viewers were invited "to make a stand, to make a statement, to make a difference" by uploading their own messages for the world to see. MadV created *The Message* out of eighty-two of these responses. "Love one another," they say. "We are all connected." "Together as one." "The human face." "One life." "*Un monde*," "one planet," "one world."

The Message is a euphoric denial of geographical distance and cultural difference. In terms of style and sentiment *BioShock* is its polar opposite, but it too offers a variation on the theme of context collapse. Unmoored from their original clinical contexts, Lumley's image and the dying man's breath become signifiers of disfigurement and abjection. They no longer possess the ability to speak of particular injuries and illnesses, or the experience of pain, endurance, or resignation. They are not "medical records" or "documentary photographs": institutional and discursive categories that belong to a less fluid world. As a source of "disturbing inspiration," the faces taken from Project Façade perform a job in the present rather than illuminating the past. There is an unfortunate irony here: the photographs taken at the Queen's Hospital record the effects of weapons that were designed to mutilate and kill. Their human subjects are redeployed within *BioShock* as targets. It is not just where historical images end up that matters, but where they began, and the distance traveled.

No consensus is reached, in the players' forum, regarding the moral rightness or wrongness of *BioShock*. The discussion thread offers a snapshot of ethical reasoning in action, as a process of working through an open-ended series of questions, rather than the application of a set of agreed principles, as in a legal code or religious text. This is clearly a situation that the game's artists and designers are comfortable with. Of course, moral ambiguity is a familiar attribute of contemporary art, and increasingly embraced by curators of nonart collections and exhibitions for whom dangerous liaisons and surprising juxtapositions are preferable to traditional didactic or aesthetic displays. In appealing to *BioShock*'s "shades of grey," the game's makers and players are aligning themselves (consciously or not) with a contemporary avant-garde that privileges uncertainty, emphasizes subjective response, questions authority and ownership—of images as well as ideas—and resists "closure."

Is *BioShock* art? If these are defining attributes, then yes, it is. But I doubt that it is the kind of art Ludmilla Jordanova was thinking of when she wrote, in her catalog essay, of the "visual pleasures that both stimulate the production of images of the body and make them of enduring fascination." The visual pleasures offered by *BioShock* are relatively uncharted waters; its powers of horror more profitable than Francis Bacon could have imagined. There is no definitive answer to the questions posed at the beginning of this chapter: what do we gain from looking at images like these, and what would constitute their proper (or improper) use? Sontag, as we have seen, emphasizes the contexts of viewing, but she also distinguishes between "photographs with the most solemn or heart-rending subject matter"—which might, in the right circumstances, serve as secular icons—and those that shock and shame us with their depiction of "real horror."[89] Unless we are in a position to do something about the suffering documented in these "extreme" images, we are simply voyeurs. Against this emotional taxonomy of images (moving versus shocking) it may be argued that "real horror" has a subjective element. Sontag's selection of most shocking photographs might not be yours or mine.

An alternative approach to such images might pay closer attention to the manifold ways in which suffering is mediated, and the circumstances under which it becomes possible to look (to *really* look) at horror. Tonks's drawings, for example, mediate and contain suffering in a way that the case photographs of the same patients cannot, but the intimacy and beauty of the drawings is not the exclusive preserve of art. There are other ways of mediating horror: through narrative or autobiography, or by formalizing the encounter between viewer and image, as in Sontag's example of the surgeon in a military hospital. Her disquiet, however, is provoked by a different kind of mediation, the "marketing of experiences, tastes and simulacra" in the name of art, education, and entertainment.[90] There seems "no way," she concludes, "to guarantee reverential conditions in which to look at these pictures and be fully responsive to them."[91] *BioShock* certainly denies us the possibility of "regarding" Lumley's pain in any meaningful sense, but it also complicates the idea of the simulacrum as a representation that replaces the real.

Within the game—as well as in the archive and the antiques and collectibles market—the value of the photographic image depends on its perceived authenticity and indexical relationship to the subject. If it turned out that the resemblance to Henry Lumley was coincidental, or that Schyman had used actors, things would be completely different. When Nias Wolf writes, "Honor the dead," I suspect that what he really means is *honor the remains of the dead.* His concern with the appropriate use of a photograph stems from the belief that photographs "capture" their subjects; that there is, magically, something of us in our likenesses. The way personhood is understood in law is very different. The Human Tissue Act, for example, works on the premise that an individual is the sum of his or her body parts. Thus defined, the "person" is protected by the legal requirement of consent. The act is silent, though, on the subject of photography and film, including clinical images and images of human remains.[92] It seems to me that Lumley and the breathing man point us toward a more dispersed understanding of personhood than that enshrined in the law: one that would encompass facial likeness and perhaps even the historical connotations of breath. If *BioShock* is unethical, it is surely because it violates a common feeling that photographs of suffering somehow contain or embody their subjects; and that they therefore carry a burden of care.

Conclusion

One of the advantages of writing academic books is that one is rarely asked to provide a personal explanation for a research interest. This project has been different. When I say that I am working on the cultural history of disfigurement, people wonder why. Looking back on the slow evolution of this book, it is clear to me now that my points of departure have been both emotional and intellectual, and inextricably so. It is *because* disfigurement is so often considered taboo that its "management" (to borrow Goffman's term) is so interesting. The same applies to the cultural framing (i.e., the management) of war and violence. These cannot *not* be personal subjects, and my own responses have inevitably informed the questions I have pursued.

The book itself has several beginnings, but one of the most decisive—because it made me aware of what I wanted to achieve—was reading Andrew Bamji's account of the developments in plastic surgery during World War I. It is fair to say that Bamji's contribution to this nascent field of study is unparalleled: my own research leans heavily on the collection of medical records, ephemera, and rare books that he assembled at Queen Mary's Hospital in Sidcup (which are now in the Royal College of Surgeons and Liddle collections). It is thanks to Bamji that there are now three novels about Harold Gillies and his patients—most famously Pat Barker's *Toby's Room*—and an international group of scholars working on the medical, social, and cultural history of facial war injuries in Britain.[1] In his article, Bamji refers to the "universal and enduring" horror of the disfigured face.[2] It is a passing observation, which I have quoted before, and serves, by way of the conclusion to his chapter, to underscore the contribution of the medical teams working at the Queen's Hospital. Thanks to them, Bamji writes, "Those disfigured by war could look forward to a better life than would otherwise have been their lot."[3]

I admit I *was* horrified when I first looked through the Sidcup files during a visit to the archive in 2005 (I remember the trip well because it was a few months before my second child was born). It seems important, however, to make a general distinction between the injured and the disfigured face. In *Regarding the Pain of Others*, Susan Sontag explores the ethics of looking at images of suffering. For the most part, the "before" photographs in the Gillies Archives are images of terrible suffering. The "after" photographs, in comparison, present a spectrum of more or less healed, more or less disfigured faces, and while scarring and loss of function could cause pain and discomfort, these are not images *of pain* in the same way. The distinction isn't absolute (some injures never healed, and for men like Henry Lumley there was no "after"); nevertheless, differentiating between injury and disfigurement makes it possible to pose a specific question: why was (and is) the *disfigured* face a source of horror? Part of the answer, I suggest in chapter 2, is that in 1914 facial disfigurement was still associated with the stigma of syphilis. Beauty and ugliness had long been regarded as the outward manifestation of moral virtue (or its lack): a set of assumptions that was compounded by the significance of the face as a site of transcendence in religious art. The available iconography of sacrifice and heroism, in other words, assumed facial integrity, legibility and beauty.

From a professional perspective, Bamji's comments are understandable: as curator of the Gillies Archives, he was primarily interested in the surgical response to facial injury. The social negotiation of stigma was secondary. His comments reflect a medical understanding of disfigurement as a treatable condition (albeit with variable results and associated risks). Iain Hutchison, one of the UK's leading maxillofacial surgeons, sums up the medical model in a sentence: "It's very distressing for me to see someone walking down the street, with a condition that's eminently treatable, who isn't seeking treatment."[4] The medical model leaves no room for what Elaine Scarry calls "the pleasure-filled tumult of staring," or the possibility of seeing anew something, or someone, formerly "confidently repudiated as an object of beauty."[5]

One of the most vocal critics of this outlook—which casts disfigurement as a personal tragedy—is James Partridge, the CEO of the British charity Changing Faces. Despite the inclusion of serious disfigurement in the Disability Discrimination Act (DDA) in 1995, Partridge worries that "the norms of acceptability are narrowing" and that society is becoming even less tolerant of people who look different from the norm: "We hoped we were going to ride a wave towards diversity and the inclusion of people with disabilities," he said in a 2007 interview, "but it's almost the other way."[6] His conviction that the "norms of acceptability" are subject to cultural and historical variation is one that I share. Like Partridge, my approach to disfigurement is grounded in a social model of disability, according to which beauty, normality, acceptability, and ugliness are in the eye (and cultural imagination) of the beholder.[7]

The writer who has most profoundly influenced my understanding of disability as social is Erving Goffman, who describes the encounter with stigma as "one of the primal scenes of sociology" because it serves to define—for a given social group, at a particular time—what it is to be fully human.[8] Goffman's concern was to elaborate the structural preconditions of stigma and its interpersonal dynamics, not its specific cultural or historical manifestations; and the experiential, self-revelatory richness of his autobiographical sources has no equivalent in the documentary record of the Great War. This poses a methodological problem for historians. How would one begin to reconstruct the *experience* of stigma, I wondered, from written sources that are so circumspect, so silent on the subject of suffering? For a time, I planned to include a chapter on stoicism, in which I would historicize the absence of emotional language in first-hand accounts of facial injury. In the end, I didn't write that chapter—although I hope someone does—because I realized that that my project was more centrally concerned with investigating the experience of the beholder. Here the primary sources were more forthcoming: from Ward Muir's *The Happy Hospital* (a paradigm of "interaction-uneasiness") to Henry Tonks's drawings (as a material record of sustained, unembarrassed looking), there are numerous accounts of the "primal scene" Goffman evokes, in which the humanity of the stigmatized individual is at stake.[9]

In keeping with my focus on the visual contexts of stigma, the historical chapters of the book explore the discourse and visibility of facial injury in wartime Britain and the United States: a subject largely neglected by historians of war and disability. Despite the considerable literature on World War I and the male body—much of it inspired by Joanna Bourke's brilliant *Dismembering the Male* (1996)—the male face has remained absent from, or at best marginal to discussions of masculinity and suffering. Yet as I have argued, facial injury and disfigurement were part of the social and cultural legacy of World War I: the way it was imagined (the "worst loss of all"); and the fantasy of repair is as relevant today as it was a century ago.

*

Another beginning: in autumn 2002, at the suggestion of my colleague Lisa Tickner, I visited the Strang Print Room at University College London to see an exhibition of Henry Tonks's surgical portraits. In art, as in photojournalism, the face is the primary signifier not just of self or identity, but of humanity (and its violation or absence is experienced as an "abyss" that marks the limits of the human). Tonks's portraits—if they can even be called that—are almost unbearably intimate studies. They have taught me something, as a historian of art, about the depths of the human face, the aesthetics of touch, and the way in which images—and institutions—can mediate the way we see. We worry about artists "aestheticizing" war or suffering, but as Sontag observes, all representations—paintings and drawings as much as documentary photographs—transform their subjects. This alchemy is what makes Tonks's surgical portraits more than medical illustrations. As an image, "Something may be beautiful—or terrifying, or unbearable, or quite bearable—as it is not in real life."[10]

Because of Tonks, this became a book about portraiture and not just a history of images of injury and their reception. None of the examples I've focused on could be described as typical portraits, though: Tonks uses the form of traditional portraiture to evoke the fragility and humanity of his patients. Wood and Ladd use it quite differently, to repair—and to hide—the war-damaged face. The contemporary examples discussed in chapter 1 are just as complex, using portraiture as a vehicle for the expression of human resilience in the face of adversity (Greenfield-Sanders, *Alive Day Memories*), and as a means of exploring the psychological and social effects of war (Berman, Griffiths). These responses indicate that the relationship between disability and aesthetics—and "disability aesthetics" and politics—is far from straightforward.

It would be impossible to conclude without mentioning Tobin Siebers's contribution to these debates. I came across his seminal and provocative book *Disability Aesthetics* (2010) several years after I had used the title "The Aesthetics of Disfigurement" in an essay on the Tonks pastels. My aim was quite specific: to work out how those drawings differed from conventional medical representations (photographs and medical illustration) and conventional portraits. My argument, which is developed in chapter 4, was that the pastels show Tonks experimenting with an aesthetics of touch. Although I used aesthetic terms (beauty, ugliness, the grotesque), my concern was to elaborate them historically and contextually—in relation to specific acts of viewing or kinds of viewers—rather than assuming a priori that I knew what they meant. I have taken the same approach to each of the case studies explored here. So it is that we find Nina Berman lighting Tyler Ziegel to make him look less "gruesome," and Stuart Griffiths sorting his photographs of Martyn Compton into "happy" shots and those that allow for a more ambiguous reading of disfigurement. For both photographers, the damaged body is a metaphor for other kinds of loss. Antiwar images like these do not look for beauty in suffering; their purpose is polemical rather than reparative.

Siebers defines "disability aesthetics" both as a critical "resource" within avant-garde modernism (the means by which traditional beauty is interrogated) and as "an aesthetic value"—a different kind of beauty, more inclusive of human variation—that is still evolving.[11] "To what concept, other than the idea of disability," he asks,

> might be referred modern art's love affair with misshapen and twisted bodies, stunning variety of human forms, intense representations of traumatic injury and psychological alienation, and unyielding preoccupation with wounds and tormented flesh?[12]

I am not sure if it matters that disability is the organizing concept here (rather than, say, "defamiliarization," "convulsive beauty," "abjection," "the Real," or "wound culture," to mention those theories most relevant to Siebers's examples).[13] For me, what matters profoundly is the invitation to think about what disability *means* and what it *does* in the context of art and visual culture, rather than simply asking whether a particular image is "right and true."[14] The contemporary examples I've looked at certainly do use the image and idea of disability as a resource: both affirmatively (as in *Alive Day Memories*) and critically (in the work of Berman and Griffiths). Siebers does not extend his analysis to horror films or computer games, but *BioShock* reveals the extent to which contemporary anxieties are—as Bryan Turner observes—"translated into disturbed images of the body."[15] Indeed, *BioShock* could be read as a satire of the medical model of disability: in their desperate pursuit of physical prowess and aesthetic perfection the citizens of Rapture have become monsters.

The historical case studies in this book are more difficult to pin down with regard to their meanings, in part because none are straightforwardly "art" and all involve some degree of censorship or curtailed visibility. Disability cannot be said to function as an aesthetic or critical "resource" for the sculptors—like Wood and Ladd—engaged in the production of portrait masks: it is something to be masked and repaired. On the other hand, the persistence of classical aesthetics makes it possible for a sculptor like Kathleen Scott to describe the ruined faces she encounters in the hospital as beautiful, "like antique marbles."[16] Is this disability as aesthetic value, or classicism as a form of sublimation? I don't know. Tonks's pastels come closest to what Siebers has in mind in their recognition of the "fragility as well as the violence of human existence,"[17] but they are not modernist or avant-garde by any stretch of the imagination. "Beauty is other today—and like no other time in human history," writes Siebers in his own conclusion. James Partridge would no doubt disagree. What is certain, though, is that Tonks's portraits have found an audience: an audience that expects art to be critical and ambiguous, and at times unbearable.

In an interview about the future of visual culture studies as an academic discipline, W. J. T. Mitchell wondered whether "the most interesting new questions . . . will be located at the frontiers of visuality, the places where seeing approaches a limit and is faced with its own negation."[18] Disfigurement is arguably one such frontier: not only because it presents us with a history of aversion (in which the act of looking is itself negated), but because the *representation* of the disfigured face disrupts the conventions of Western art, and by extension, a whole pictorial language of identity and empathy. Most of the historical photographs and drawings reproduced in these pages were not part of the public visual culture of the Great War. They might move us, today, to contemplate the futility of war or the magnitude of individual sacrifice, but commemoration was never their intended purpose. Because many of these images originated in a clinical context, they occupy an ethical borderland in which legal definitions of privacy, personhood, and human rights compete with the contemporary politics of witnessing, memory, and memorialization: a space of fantasy where fascination and aversion are found in equal measure.

Notes

Introduction

1. Holland Cotter, "Words Unspoken Are Rendered on War's Faces," *New York Times*, August 22, 2007, http://www.nytimes.com/2007/08/22/arts/design/22berm.html, accessed June 19, 2016.

2. Nina Berman, "The Face of War," interview by Lindsay Beyerstein, *Salon.com*, March 10, 2007, http://www.salon.com/life/feature/2007/03/10/berman_photo, accessed June 19, 2016.

3. Berman, "The Face of War."

4. From Nina Berman's interview by Richard Bradley, "Nina Berman at Last," posted June 8, 2010, http://www.richardbradley.net/shotsinthe-dark/2010/06/08/6731/, accessed June 19, 2016.

5. Sontag, *Regarding the Pain of Others*, 6.

6. Woolf, *Three Guineas*, 10.

7. Woolf, *Three Guineas*, 10.

8. Turner, "Social Fluids," 1, 6.

9. Biernoff, *Sight and Embodiment.*

10. This was a recurring theme in the responses to the *October* questionnaire on visual culture, *October* 77, "Visual Culture" special issue (Summer 1996): 25–70.

11. See, for example, Carden-Coyne, *Reconstructing the Body*; Das, *Touch and Intimacy in First World War Literature*; Koureas, *Memory, Masculinity and National Identity*; and Meyer, *Men of War*. There have been parallel developments in the historiography of disability and rehabilitation. The most relevant texts are Cooter, *Surgery and Society*; Koven, "Remembering and Dismemberment"; Gerber, *Disabled Veterans*; Cohen, *The War Came Home*; Reznick, *Healing the Nation*; and Linker, *War's Waste.*

12. Carden-Coyne, *Reconstructing the Body*, 4.

13. Carden-Coyne, *Reconstructing the Body*, 5.

14. The original source is Fielding H. Garrison, *Notes on the History of Military Medicine* (1922). Carden-Coyne, *Reconstructing the Body*, 70–71.

15. Carden-Coyne, *Reconstructing the Body*, 87.

16. War art and photography are discussed more briefly, perhaps because they have received sustained attention elsewhere. Sue Malvern's *Modern Art, Britain and the Great War* and Paul Gogh's *A Terrible Beauty* are the most comprehensive studies of the British war artists; the standard texts on World War I photography are Carmichael, *First World War Photographers*; and Taylor, *War Photography*.

17. Carden-Coyne, *Reconstructing the Body*, 108.

18. I have borrowed the term "throw" from Mandler, "The Problem with Cultural History."

19. Quoted in Carmichael, *First World War Photographers*, 34–35.

20. Das, *Touch and Intimacy*, 7.

21. Carden-Coyne, *Reconstructing the Body*, 15.

22. Bourke, *Dismembering the Male*, 12.

23. Bourke, *Dismembering the Male*, 12.

24. See, for example, the UK Office for Disability Issues website: http://odi.dwp.gov.uk/about-the-odi/the-social-model.php, accessed December 17, 2013.

25. Davis, "Introduction: Normality, Power, and Culture," 1.

26. Wardle and Boyce, "Media Coverage and Audience Reception," summary, n.p.

27. Wardle and Boyce, "Media Coverage and Audience Reception," summary, n.p.

28. Bourke, *Dismembering the Male*, 15, 33.

29. See Koureas, *Memory, Masculinity and National Identity*, 138–42.

30. Carden-Coyne, *Reconstructing the Body*, 60, 96–103.

31. Turner, *Body and Society*, 7–8, quoted in Fraser and Greco, *The Body*, 33.

32. Sekula, "Body and the Archive," 6–7; Fraser and Greco, *The Body*, 164.

33. Sekula, "Body and the Archive," 10.

34. The "archival promise" of photography was, however, gradually frustrated by "the messy contingency of the photograph" and "the sheer quantity of images" (Sekula, "Body and the Archive," 17). Sekula contrasts this "older" (physiognomic/photographic) model of "optical truth" to the "abstract" statistical methods that characterize sociopolitical and scientific discourse in the twentieth century (55).

35. Foucault, *Discipline and Punish*, 200–201.

36. Sekula, "Body and the Archive," 7.

37. Sekula, "Body and the Archive," 10.

38. Johann Caspar Lavater's four-volume work *Essays on Physiognomy* (1775–78) was largely responsible for the resurgence of interest in physiognomy in Western Europe. Lavater's sources included Aristotle, Plato, and Della Porta's *De Humana Physiognomonia* (1586).

39. Sekula, "Body and the Archive," 12.

40. Sennett, *The Fall of Public Man*, 171.

41. The term "perceptual agenda" is from Twine, "Physiognomy."

42. Gillies quoted in Bamji, "Facial Surgery," 495.

43. "As the face with us is chiefly admired for its beauty," observed Charles Darwin in *The Descent of Man*, "so with savages it is the chief seat of mutilation." Quoted in Gilman, *Making the Body Beautiful*, xviii.

44. "Death by disfigurement" is well illustrated on the wiki *TV Tropes*, "a catalog of the tricks of the trade for writing fiction." http://tvtropes.org/pmwiki/pmwiki.php/Main/DeathByDisfigurement, accessed October 3, 2012.

45. Orlan in Fraser and Greco, *The Body*, 312–13.

46. Orlan, quoted in Hirschhorn, "Orlan," 126.

47. On the history of before-and-after photography, see Gilman, *Making the Body Beautiful*, 36–42.

48. Orlan, in Fraser and Greco, *The Body*, 314.

49. Adams, *Emptiness of the Image*, 154.

50. Orlan, in an interview with the Australian radio presenter Phillip Adams on "Late Night Live," ABC Radio National, December 8, 1992.

51. Barthes, *A Lover's Discourse*, 73.

52. From Nina Berman's interview by Richard Bradley, "Nina Berman at Last," posted June 10, 2010, http://www.richardbradley.net/shotsinthedark/2010/06/10/nina-berman-part-2/, accessed June 19, 2016.

53. Gilman, *Making the Body Beautiful*, 23.

54. Gilman, *Making the Body Beautiful*, 168.

55. Gilman, *Making the Body Beautiful*, 162.

56. The key sources are Aristotle's *Generation of Animals* (ca. 350 BCE), Cicero's *On Divination* (44 BCE), and Pliny the Elder's *Natural History* (first century CE).

57. Medieval scholars referred to Augustine's discussion of monstrous births in *The City of God*, xxi.8 (early fifth century) and Isidore of Seville's commentary in the *Etymologies*, xi.3 (ca. 630).

58. *The Opus Majus of Roger Bacon*, vol. 2: 672.

59. Park and Daston, "Unnatural Conceptions," 23.

60. Garland-Thomson, *Freakery*.

61. Garland-Thomson, *Freakery*, 2.

62. David Hume, *An Enquiry Concerning Human Understanding*, quoted in Park and Daston, "Unnatural Conceptions," 54.

63. Bogdan, "Social Construction of Freaks," 34.

64. Two particularly influential examples of this literature are Mary Russo's *The Female Grotesque* and Stallybrass and White, *The Politics and Poetics of Transgression*.

65. The book had its origins in Bakhtin's dissertation on Rabelais, which he completed in 1940.

66. Bakhtin, *Rabelais*, in Fraser and Greco, *The Body*, 92.

67. Bakhtin regarded the classical and the grotesque as oppositional "canons" that are not, however, necessarily discrete or immutable (*Rabelais*, 30).

68. Bakhtin, *Rabelais*, in Fraser and Greco, *The Body*, 93.

69. Bakhtin, *Rabelais*, in Fraser and Greco, *The Body*, 95.

70. Muir, *The Happy Hospital*, 143–44.

71. Shaw, "Disgusting Objects."

72. On Civil War medical photographs, see Connor and Rhode, "Shooting Soldiers"; Davis, "A Terrible Distinctiveness"; and Newman, "Wounds and Wounding."

73. "A War Museum in Paris," *Times* (London), April 9, 1917, 9.

74. Albert G. Bettman, "The Psychology of Appearances," *Northwest Medicine* 28 (1929): 184, quoted in Gilman, *Making the Body Beautiful*, 161. See also Pound, *Gillies*, 39.

75. "Miracles They Work at Frognal," *Daily Sketch*, April 1918. London Metropolitan Archives, HO2/QM/Y01/05.

76. For a discussion of the politics and aesthetics of trauma in Weimar Germany, see Fox, "Confronting Post-war Shame."

77. Corbett, *The Modernity of English Art*, 1.

78. Muir, *Happy Hospital*, 144.

79. Lady Kennet [Kathleen, Lady Scott], *Self-Portrait of an Artist*, entry for October 19, 1918, 167.

80. Further biographical details are given in Crellin, "Hollow Men"; Mitchell, "Facing Horror"; and Romm and Zacher, "Anna Coleman Ladd."

81. The film is in the Wellcome Library, and on several websites including the *Smithsonian Magazine:* http://www.smithsonianmag.com/history-archaeology/mask.html, accessed December 30, 2010.

82. *Henry Tonks: Art and Surgery*, University College London, October 2, 2002—March 28, 2003. Gillies Archives image collection: http://www.gilliesarchives.org.uk/Tonks%20pastels/index.html, accessed December 30, 2010.

83. *Faces of Battle* was the culmination of the Wellcome Trust–funded Project Façade: http://www.projectfacade.com, accessed June 10, 2009.

84. *Faces of Battle*, for example, presented graphic documentation of facial injury alongside interpretive textile sculptures by the artist and curator Paddy Hartley.

85. Winter, *Sites of Memory*, 172, 225–26.

86. Kristeva, *Black Sun*, 24–25.

87. Winter, *Sites of Memory*, 226–27.

88. "Forms of aesthetic redemption" is Winter's phrase. *Sites of Memory*, 225.

89. Referring to literary and religious representation, Kristeva writes: "If psychoanalysts think they are more efficacious, notably through strengthening the subject's cognitive possibilities, they also owe it to themselves to enrich their practice by paying greater attention to these sublimatory solutions to our crises, in order to be lucid counterdepressants rather than neutralising antidepressants." *Black Sun*, 25.

90. Paul Nash, describing the western front in a letter to his wife Margaret, November 13–16, 1917, reprinted in Nash, *Outline*, 210.

91. "Surveying the interstices of art and medicine, death and culture" is the tagline of Joanna Ebenstein's popular *Morbid Anatomy* blog, http://morbidanatomy.blogspot.co.uk/, accessed June 19, 2016.

92. Garland-Thomson, *Freakery*, 1.

93. Garland-Thomson, *Staring*, 10.

94. Garland-Thomson, *Staring*, 9–10.

95. Garland-Thomson, *Staring*, 45.

96. Garland-Thomson, *Staring*, 19, paraphrasing Turner, *Vulnerability*.

97. "There is probably no area of contemporary life in which some idea of a norm, mean, or average has not been calculated," notes Lennard J. Davis in his introduction to *The Disability Studies Reader*, 1.

98. Garland-Thomson, *Staring*, 20.

99. "Meet the Superhumans" was the tagline of the Channel 4 media campaign, July 18, 2012, http://www.channel4.com/info/press/news/channel-4-takes-over-tv-with-meet-the-superhumans-campaign, accessed June 20, 2016.

100. Garland-Thomson, *Staring*, 9, 185, 198 n.9.

101. Garland-Thomson, *Staring*, 50–51, 188–89.

102. Garland-Thomson, *Staring*, 81.

103. Garland-Thomson, *Staring*, 188.

Chapter 1

1. Butler, *Precarious Life*, 146.

2. http://icasualties.org/OEF/Index.aspx, accessed December 4, 2012. The reporting of Afghan casualties did not begin until 2007: for estimates see Susan G.

Chesser, *Afghanistan Casualties: Military Forces and Civilians*, Congressional Research Service, September 6, 2012, www.fas.org/sgp/crs/natsec/R41084.pdf, accessed June 20, 2016.

3. "Seven Years in Iraq," *Time* online, March 19, 2010, http://www.time.com/time/specials/packages/article/0,28804,1967340_1967378_1968135,00.html, accessed December 4, 2012.

4. The Western media's failure to adequately represent these events has been widely remarked upon by analysts of embedded journalism. See, for example, Katovsky and Carlson, *Embedded*; Stallabrass, *Memory of Fire*; and Seib, *Beyond the Front Lines*.

5. Carmichael, *First World War Photographers*, 1–2.

6. The president of the Military Reporters and Editors Association, Sig Christenson, gives the somewhat lower figure of 570 embedded journalists in "The Vanishing Embedded Reporter in Iraq," *Journalism.org*, October 26, 2006, http://www.journalism.org/node/2596, accessed June 19, 2016.

7. Stallabrass, *Memory of Fire*, 35.

8. Michael Kamber, Battlespace project, audio recording: http://www.battlespaceonline.org/#, accessed July 8, 2013.

9. Dan Kennedy, "Iraq's Unseen Violence," *Guardian*, July 29, 2008, https://www.theguardian.com/commentisfree/2008/jul/29/iraqandthemedia.usa, accessed June 20, 2016.

10. The U.S. media blackout on showing the flag-draped coffins of the returning war dead was not lifted until April 2009, after Obama took office and reversed the ban imposed in 1991 during the lead-up to the Gulf War.

11. "Bloodless and anodyne" is Stallabrass's description, *Memory of Fire*, 41.

12. Nessen et al., *War Surgery in Afghanistan and Iraq*.

13. Sue Halpern, "The War We Don't Want to See," *New York Review*, December 18, 2008, 60–62.

14. I have borrowed the term "heroic individualism" from Apel, *War Culture and the Contest of Images*, Kindle edition, loc. 1953–54.

15. Turner, review of *Alive Day Memories*, 289.

16. Interview with James Gandolfini on the HBO Alive Day Memories website, http://www.hbo.com/documentaries/alive-day-memories-home-from-iraq/index.html#/documentaries/alive-day-memories-home-from-iraq/interview/james-gandolfini.html, accessed April 30, 2013.

17. Nevins, quoted in Bill Carter, "The Price of War, Front and Center," *New York Times*, September 6, 2007, http://www.nytimes.com/2007/09/06/arts/06iht-07hbo.7404924.html?pagewanted=all&_r=0, accessed April 30, 2013.

18. Nevins, quoted in Carter, "Price of War," n.p.

19. Schick, quoted in Carter, "Price of War," n.p.

20. Jones, quoted in Carter, "Price of War," n.p.

21. Gandolfini, quoted in Carter, "Price of War," n.p.

22. Nevins, quoted in Carter, "Price of War," n.p.

23. "Repairing war's ravages: renovating facial injuries" is the caption that accompanies Horace Nicholls's photographs of facial reconstruction in the Imperial War Museum, London. UCLA's Operation Mend is a recent example of this discourse of repair.

24. Turner, review of *Alive Day Memories*, 289.

25. *NBC Nightly News*, September 5, 2007, http://www.youtube.com/watch?v=mstpgpe070U, accessed May 14, 2013.

26. Gandolfini, quoted in Carter, "Price of War," n.p.

27. Turner, review of *Alive Day Memories*, 289.

28. Butler, *Frames of War*, 3.

29. Butler, *Frames of War*, 29.

30. Butler, *Frames of War*, 67. Photographs can move and challenge us, Sontag argues, but they don't on their own produce understanding or motivate political action. Sontag, *Regarding the Pain of Others*, 80.

31. Butler, *Frames of War*, 11, 100 (my italics).

32. Apel, *War Culture*, Kindle edition, loc. 1954.

33. Apel, *War Culture*, Kindle edition, loc. 1953.

34. Vetrocq, "Rules of Engagement," 175.

35. Vetrocq, "Rules of Engagement," 175.

36. Peter Applebome, "Soldiers' Portraits Make the Costs of War More Visible," *New York Times*, September 27, 2007, http://www.nytimes.com/2007/09/27/nyregion/27towns.html, accessed May 25, 2013.

37. Dawn Halfaker, HBO Alive Day Memories interview, YouTube, http://www.youtube.com/watch?v=mCZ4XJx-lJs, accessed April 25, 2013.

38. Apel, *War Culture*, Kindle edition, loc. 1964.

39. "My Turn: Nina Berman," audio recording, Whitney Biennial events program, May 28, 2010, http://whitney.org/WatchAndListen/Tag?context=biennial&play_id=95, accessed June 19, 2016.

40. Berman, *Homeland*.

41. "My Turn: Nina Berman."

42. Noor / Nina Berman, *Purple Hearts*, http://vimeo.com/48285708, accessed June 10, 2013.

43. Verlyn Klinkenborg, introduction to Berman, *Purple Hearts*.

44. Stuart Griffiths, interviewed during the 2010 Brighton Photo Fringe, http://www.youtube.com/watch?v=7MpmQf4NCmQ, accessed July 19, 2013.

45. Stuart Griffiths, interviewed by Patrick Butler, "On Civvy Streets," *Guardian* Society supplement, May 4, 2005, http://www.guardian.co.uk/society/2005/may/04/homelessness.guardiansocietysupplement, accessed October 29, 2010.

46. Stuart Griffiths, "The Soldier's Tale: Return from Iraq," *Independent*, March 16, 2008, http://www.independent.co.uk/news/uk/this-britain/the-soldiers-tale-return-from-iraq-795524.html, accessed December 28, 2010.

47. Sneersnipe film review, http://www.sneersnipe.co.uk/review_title.php?id=519, accessed June 27, 2013.

48. Conversation with the author, October 8, 2010.

49. Julian Stallabrass, "The Power and Impotence of Images," in *Memory of Fire*, 48.

50. Van Alphen, "The Portrait's Dispersal."

51. "[*Alive Day Memories*] puts a face to some of the many soldiers and Marines who've come back in record numbers suffering from severe injuries and trauma, and who, in many ways, have been hidden from the public's view." HBO website, accessed April 30, 2013.

52. Butler, *Precarious Life*, 141.

53. Butler, *Precarious Life*, 142.

54. "War/Photography: An Interview with Simon Norfolk," on *BLDGBLOG*, November 2006, http://bldgblog.blogspot.co.uk/2006/11/warphotography-interview-with-simon.html, quoted in James, "Making an Ugly World Beautiful," 125.

55. Stallabrass, *Memory of Fire*, 54.

56. Stallabrass, *Memory of Fire*, 54.

57. James, "Making an Ugly World Beautiful," 125.

58. Jordanova, *Defining Features*, 20.

59. Van Alphen, "The Portrait's Dispersal."

60. Bourdieu, *Distinction*, 190–208.

61. I have taken this phrase from Van Alphen, "The Portrait's Dispersal," 239.

62. From Berman's interview by Richard Bradley, "Nina Berman at Last," June 10, 2010, *Shots in the Dark*, http://www.richardbradley.net/shotsinthedark/2010/06/10/nina-berman-part-2/, accessed June 19, 2016. The most balanced account of Ziegel in the press is Ariel Leve, "Tyler Ziegel and Renee: One Year On," *Sunday Times*, May 11, 2008, http://www.timesonline.co.uk/tol/news/world/us_and_americas/article3886348.ece, accessed December 30, 2010. Leve visited the couple with Berman.

63. Goffman, *Stigma*, 11.

64. Goffman, *Stigma*, 11.

65. Peirce, "Logic as Semiotic," 109. Cf. Johansen, *Signs in Use*, 32.

66. Goffman, *Stigma*, 14, 163–64.

67. Goffman, *Stigma*, 14.

68. Although the term "disability" is associated with functional impairment and "deformity" implies a purely physical deviation of form, both have the potential to impair social interaction in the presence of stigma (a point to which we will return in chapters 3 and 4).

69. Goffman, *Stigma*, 16.

70. Simi Linton, "Blind People and Other Spurious Tales," *Disability Culture Watch*, November 30, 2007, http://similinton.com/blog/?p=92, accessed November 7, 2011.

71. Goffman, *Stigma*, 14.

72. Berman, "Nina Berman at Last."

73. Goffman, *Stigma*, 30.

74. Interview with Stuart Griffiths, November 22, 2010.

75. Marianna Proietti was the first woman soldier below the rank of officer to be sent to the Gulf in 1991 as a member of the Royal Army Medical Corps.

76. Iversen et al., "Risk Factors for Post-traumatic Stress Disorder."

77. Interview with Stuart Griffiths, November 22, 2010.

78. Interview with Stuart Griffiths, November 22, 2010.

79. Interview with Stuart Griffiths, November 22, 2010.

80. *Closer* was first shown at the 2010 Brighton Photo Fringe, where it won the Open award, and subsequently exhibited at London College of Communication (May 3–17, 2013).

81. Interview with Stuart Griffiths, November 22, 2010.

82. Interview with Stuart Griffiths, November 22, 2010.

83. Foucault, *The Birth of the Clinic*.

84. Michelle Clifford, quoted in Angela Levin, "The Most Beautiful Wedding of the Year as Scarred Soldier Marries His Sweetheart," *Mail Online*, last modified July 14, 2008, http://www.dailymail.co.uk/femail/article-1034570/The-beautiful-wedding-year-scarred-soldier-marries-sweetheart.html, accessed June 19, 2016.

85. Levin, "The most Beautiful Wedding of the Year."

86. Interview with Stuart Griffiths, November 22, 2010.

87. Levin, "The Most Beautiful Wedding of the Year."

88. Linda Nochlin, "Some Women Realists," *Arts Magazine*, May 1974, 29, quoted in Van Alphen, "The Portrait's Dispersal," 239.

89. Stuart Griffiths, "The Soldier's Tale," *Independent*, March 16, 2008.

90. Vetrocq, "Rules of Engagement," 175.

91. Vetrocq, "Rules of Engagement," 208.

92. Wehbi, "Representing Disability and Disfigurement," accessed November 21, 2012.

93. "My Turn: Nina Berman."

94. "My Turn: Nina Berman."

95. "My Turn: Nina Berman." See also Berman's interview with Bárbara Coutinho for the Lisbon Consortium Summer School 2011, http://www.youtube.com/watch?v=LC16wwLjEOA&list=PL2D925F0C6AFBFA91, accessed July 29, 2013.

96. Berman made a short film incorporating stills and interviews from *Purple Hearts* for the 2010 Whitney Biennial, Vimeo, http://vimeo.com/15756887, accessed June 19, 2016.

97. "My Turn: Nina Berman."

98. Lisbon Consortium interview.

99. Lisbon Consortium interview.

100. Apel, *War Culture*, Kindle edition, loc. 2032.

101. Berman, quoted in the *New York Times' Lens* blog, "Showcase: The War's Long Shadows," June 11, 2009, http://lens.blogs.nytimes.com/2009/06/11/showcase-3/, accessed June 19, 2016.

102. mad@er, June 9, 2010, (5:31 p.m.), comment on Berman's interview by Richard Bradley, "Nina Berman at Last."

103. As Berman says to Richard Bradley: "What's art, what is the place for journalism?" "Nina Berman: The Conclusion," June 11, 2010, *Shots in the Dark*, http://www.richardbradley.net/shotsinthedark/2010/06/11/nina-berman-the-conclusion/, accessed June 19, 2016.

104. Butler, *Precarious Life*, 144–45.

105. Butler, *Precarious Life*, 144.

106. For a discussion of the historical permutations of "likeness," see Woodall, introduction to *Portraiture: Facing the Subject*, 1–25.

Chapter 2

1. Service, *Rhymes of a Red Cross Man*, 54.

2. Bourke, *Dismembering the Male*, 33. Harold Gillies's surgical team had performed 11,572 major facial operations by the time the war ended. Pound, *Gillies*, 54.

3. Bamji, "Facial Surgery," 495. Gillies and Millard, *Principles and Art of Plastic Surgery*, vol. 1: 45.

4. Albee, *A Surgeon's Fight to Rebuild Men*. Albee was famous for revolutionizing bone-grafting techniques in orthopedic as well as facial surgery.

5. *Faces of Battle*, November 2007–August 2008, National Army Museum, London.

6. Apel, "Cultural Battlegrounds." Popular illustrated histories included *The War Budget*, *The War Illustrated*, and *T.P.'s Journal of Great Deeds of the Great War* (which was published from the offices of the *Daily Telegraph*). Newnes's *The War of the Nations*, and *The Great War* (Amalgamated Press), also contained visual material. Published retrospectively in annual volumes, *The Times History of the War* is the most authoritative account.

7. Sandy Callister makes a similar point about the New Zealand context, remark-

ing that images of facial injury have been "conspicuously absent from our nation's war historiography." Callister, "Broken Gargoyles," 112.

8. "Always look a man straight in the face," one sister told her staff. Macdonald, *Roses of No Man's Land*, 149–50.

9. Muir, *Happy Hospital*, 143.

10. See, for example, Cooter, "War and Modern Medicine"; Koven, "Remembering and Dismemberment"; Bourke, *Dismembering the Male*, 31–75; Gerber, *Disabled Veterans*, which includes chapters by Cohen and Reznick; Cohen, *The War Came Home*; Guyatt, "Better Legs"; Perry, "Re-arming the Disabled Veteran"; Reznick, "Prostheses and Propaganda" and *Healing the Nation*; and Linker, *War's Waste*.

11. Gilman, *Making the Body Beautiful*, 162.

12. Cole, *About Face*, 2.

13. Merleau-Ponty, *The Primacy of Perception*, 146.

14. Muir, *Happy Hospital*, 145.

15. "Surgical Marvels: Restoring the Men Who Went Over the Top. A National Appeal," *Sunday Chronicle*, June 1918. LMA, HO2/QM/Y01/05.

16. Henry Tonks file, Imperial War Museum, London, item 18, August 18, 1917.

17. Although the arsenic-containing antibiotic Salvarsan had been used with some success since 1909, there was no effective cure for advanced syphilis until penicillin became widely available after World War II.

18. Kristeva, *Black Sun*, 24–25. Winter (*Sites of Memory*, 225–27) draws inspiration from Kristeva's account of "symbolic collapse" and its "sublimatory solutions" (which Kristeva sees as aesthetic and religious as well as psychoanalytic). In this sense, the surgical and prosthetic reconstruction of faces could be seen as continuous with the broader tendencies Winter identifies in visual and material culture. Veterans' bodies, too, were contested sites of bereavement and commemoration; of "symbolic collapse" and attempted sublimation.

19. Bamji, "Facial Surgery," 500.

20. Bamji, "Facial Surgery," 495–96.

21. Bourke, *Dismembering the Male*, 213.

22. The original painting by James Clark was donated to a war relief charity and bought by Queen Mary for Princess Beatrice, in memory of her son Prince Maurice of Battenberg, who died at Ypres. It now hangs in the Battenberg Chapel, St Mildred's Church, on the Isle of Wight. Paul Breen, "The Art of Sacrifice," March 31, 2010, IWM War Memorials Archive Blog, http://ukniwm.wordpress.com/tag/ww1/. UK National Inventory of War Memorials, http://www.ukniwm.org.uk/server/show/conMemorial.59639/fromUkniwmSearch/1, accessed September 19, 2013.

23. T. W. Pym and Geoffrey Gordon, *Papers from Picardy by Two Chaplains* (London, 1917), 175–76, quoted in Bourke, *Dismembering the Male*, 212.

24. "No feature of the war has been more striking than the religious feeling it has evolved," begins an editorial in the *Times* (October 4, 1914, 3). "War is a supreme test of reality," the author continues, "and nothing in man is more real than the instinct that urges him to sacrifice himself for an ideal which to him is dearer than life itself."

25. Bourke, *Dismembering the Male*, 248.

26. Arthur Graeme West, *The Diary of a Dead Officer: Being the Posthumous Papers of Arthur Graeme West* (London, 1918), 67, quoted in Bourke, *Dismembering the Male*, 213.

27. The print in the Wellcome Library is 32.7 × 45.3 cm. Ref. ICV No 16016.

28. Kristeva, "Holbein's Dead Christ," in *Black Sun*, 105–38.

29. Dostoyevsky, *The Idiot*, 236, 418–20.

30. Koureas, *Memory, Masculinity and National Identity,* 186.

31. Sontag, *Illness as Metaphor,* 126.

32. Sontag, *Illness as Metaphor,* 125.

33. Karl Rosenkranz, introduction to *The Aesthetics of Ugliness,* quoted in Eco, *Ugliness,* 256.

34. Eco, *Ugliness,* 16. Eco's companion anthology *On Beauty* was published in 2010.

35. Eco, *Ugliness,* 16.

36. Rosenkranz, quoted in Eco, *Ugliness,* 16.

37. Quoted in Gilman, *Making the Body Beautiful,* 51.

38. Hutchinson, *Syphilis,* 458–60, quoted in Gilman, *Making the Body Beautiful,* 50.

39. Leroux, *The Phantom of the Opera,* 12.

40. Gilman, *Making the Body Beautiful,* 52.

41. Bamji, "Facial Surgery," 499. For additional biographical information on Gillies's patients, see Bamji, "The Art of Medicine."

42. "So the resolute men fight on, suffering, tormented, maimed; but their teeth are set and the light in their eyes is high, and never does their agony debase them." "Laughing in the Face of Pain: The Fortitude of the Wounded," *T.P.'s Journal of Great Deeds of the Great War,* vol. 2, March 6, 1915, 216.

43. "Laughing in the Face of Pain," 215.

44. As listed in the *Bexley Heath Observer,* November 1921.

45. Liddle Collection, University of Leeds. The essays are cataloged as Wounds, Item 34:6, with the note "Narratives by Badly Wounded Soldiers, 'My Personal Experiences and Reminiscences of the Great War,' Collected by Lady Gough at Sidcup Hospital, 1922. Written for an education class."

46. From the essay by Private Gillimore, Second Gloucestershire Regiment.

47. The psychological rehabilitation of British servicemen of World War I with facial injuries is discussed by Millar, who comments that there are "no signs of regret or despair" in the essays written at Sidcup ("Almost Forgotten Men," 22).

48. Best was a Private in the Second Battalion Royal Scots and was wounded in the cheek at Ypres in September 1914 after only a few days of action.

49. Liddle Collection, GS 0790, Holtzapffel, J.G.H. Typescript recollections, 80.

50. Holtzapffel typescript, 81.

51. Holtzapffel typescript, 82.

52. In 1920 the building was leased by the National Institute for the Blind and became the new home of St Dunstan's Hostel. "Lost Hospitals of London," updated April 2009, http://ezitis.myzen.co.uk/sirjohnellerman.html, accessed June 19, 2016.

53. Holtzapffel's impressions can be contrasted with those of John Glubb, a young officer wounded in the face at Arras, who spent three months at the Third London General Hospital toward the end of 1917. During his stay, he wrote in memoir, "No doctor ever looked at our wounds or removed the bandages." He was finally transferred to the new hospital for facial injuries at Sidcup in Kent, where he was treated by Harold Gillies. Glubb, *Into Battle,* 193.

54. Holtzapffel typescript, 84.

55. Lady Kennet, *Self-Portrait of an Artist,* 168.

56. On the history of "convalescent blues," see Reznick, *Healing the Nation,* chap. 5.

57. Holtzapffel typescript, 84.

58. Holtzapffel typescript, 87.

59. G. E. Whitfield, Capt. to Mrs Evans, February 16, 1916. Liddle Collection, GS 1816, Evans, Reginald J.T., box 1.

60. Letter dated March 10, 1916. Liddle Collection, GS 1816, Evans, Reginald J.T., box 1.

61. Letter dated March 18, 1916. Liddle Collection, GS 1816, Evans, Reginald J.T., box 1.

62. Letter dated April 9, 1916. Liddle Collection, GS 1816, Evans, Reginald J.T., box 1.

63. Letter dated April 14, 1916. Liddle Collection, GS 1816, Evans, Reginald J.T., box 1.

64. Bamji, "The Art of Medicine," 718.

65. "Worst Loss of All," *Manchester Evening Chronicle*, press clipping dated May–June 1918, LMA.

66. Muir's prewar publications include *The Amazing Mutes* (1910); *When We Are Rich* (1911); and *Cupid's Caterers* (1914).

67. Muir, *Happy Hospital*, 143–44.

68. The program, dated December 19, 1919, is in the Gillies Archives.

69. Other injuries in this category were "loss of two or more limbs, loss of an arm and an eye, loss of a leg and an eye, loss of both hands or all fingers and thumbs, loss of both feet, loss of a hand or a foot, total loss of sight, total paralysis, lunacy, wounds or disease resulting in a man being permanently bedridden, wounds to internal organs or head involving total permanent disability." Table of war pensions for physical injury, Ministry of Pensions leaflet, ca. 1920, reproduced in Bourke, *Dismembering the Male*, 66.

70. Bourke, *Dismembering the Male*, 65.

71. Bourke, *Dismembering the Male*, 67.

72. Shilling, *Body and Social Theory*, 140; Bourdieu, *Distinction*, 190–208.

73. Gillies, *Plastic Surgery of the Face*, vii.

74. Muir, *Observations of an Orderly*, 88.

75. "Worst Loss of All," *Manchester Evening Chronicle*, May–June 1918.

76. "Moulding New Faces," *Daily Mail*, September 15, 1916. Quoted in Pound, *Gillies*, 39. Variations on this theme can be found in the newspaper clippings held at the LMA, HO2/QM/Y01/05.

77. Nurse Black's story is relayed by Gillies, *Principles and Art of Plastic Surgery*, 8. Further examples are cited by Lubin, "Masks, Mutilation and Modernity," 8.

78. Albee, *A Surgeon's Fight*, 110.

79. LMA, HO2/QM/Y01/05.

80. "The Loneliest of All Tommies," *Sunday Herald*, June 1918; "Miracles They Work at Frognal," *Daily Sketch*, April 1918.

81. "Facial Surgery for Sailors and Soldiers," *Morning Post*, July 1917.

82. "Miracles," *Daily Sketch*, April 1918. Patients at The Queen's Hospital were free to leave the estate during the day: along the road into Sidcup there were reserved benches, painted blue, so that they would not have to sit next to members of the public. Bamji, "Facial Surgery," 498. There are several anecdotes concerning disfigured veterans in Nicolson's *The Great Silence*, 61–68.

83. "Queen and Our Wounded: New Special Hospital," *Morning Post*, January 1917; "Facial Injuries: New Soldiers' Hospital in Kent," *Times* (London), January 1917.

84. "A 'Roehampton' for Facial Injuries," *Guardian*, August 1917.

85. Albert G. Bettman, "The Psychology of Appearances," *Northwest Medicine* 28 (1929): 184, quoted in Gilman, *Making the Body Beautiful*, 161. See also Pound, *Gillies*, 39.

86. "Our Hospital Page," *Daily Graphic*, July 1917.

87. Liddle Collection, GS 0790, Holtzapffel, J.G.H. Undated press clipping (ca. 1920).

88. "The Queen's Hospital," *Kent Messenger*, August 1917. The same story appears in the *Morning Post*, July 1917.

89. The visit of the queen and princesses to an exhibition of toys, beadwork, and woodwork made by patients at Sidcup is reported in the *Times*, December 9, 1919, 11. The queen chose a small gray chimpanzee as a souvenir.

90. J. Hodgson Lobley, *The Queen's Hospital for Facial Injuries, Frognal, Sidcup: The Toy Makers' Shop*, ca. 1918. Oil on canvas, 45 × 60.7 cm. Imperial War Museum, ART 3756.

91. Pound, *Gillies*, 35. One of the roles of the nursing staff at Sidcup (which included Gillies's wife Kathleen) was to "revive hope in despairing hearts." Pound notes that depression was a particular problem "when the repair work failed" (46–47).

92. McKenzie, *Reclaiming the Maimed*, 117. The Canadian-born physician was celebrated as much for his sculptures of athletes and love of scouting as for his contribution to physical education and therapy.

93. "Music in the Wards," *Evening Standard*, June 1918.

94. *The Times History of the War*, vol. 7: 344.

95. "New Limbs for Old," *Daily Mail*, August 1916.

96. The term "disabled warriors" is from the *Daily Sketch*, November 1915, accompanying a photograph of "war-time golf." This and similar articles can be found in the press clippings file from Queen Mary's Hospital (Roehampton) May 1915–February 1917, held at the LMA, HO2/QM/Y01/01. In *The Times History of the War* (vol. 13: 343–60), Roehampton is described as "a place of pilgrimage because of the wonderful results obtained there."

97. For example, the *Evening News* and *Lloyd's Weekly News*, September 1916.

98. Bourke, *Dismembering the Male*, 59; "The Disabled Soldier," *Liverpool Chronicle*, June 27, 1917, quoted in Bourke, 58.

99. Galsworthy, *Handbook for the Limbless*, vi.

100. This was the theme of the Eugenics Society's Galton Anniversary address in February 1917. Darwin, "The Disabled Sailor and Soldier."

101. Guyatt, "Better Legs," 320.

102. Figure 22 was subsequently reprinted in *The Times History of the War*, vol. 13 (345) to illustrate the care of disabled British soldiers.

103. For a comparison of the treatment and experiences of disabled ex-servicemen in Britain and Germany, see Cohen, *The War Come Home*.

104. Galsworthy, *Reveille*, 10, 15. Previously published under the title *Recalled to Life*, the quarterly journal for wounded servicemen acquired a broader remit under Galsworthy's editorship: "to reveal what the work of restoration means, to those who are being restored, to those restoring them, but even more—to the nation at large" (3).

105. Koven, "Remembering and Dismemberment," 1191.

106. Bourke, *Dismembering the Male*, 74. "Prejudice flourished," notes Bourke, citing the popular belief that disabled ex-servicemen were likely to produce crippled or limbless children. The "curious belief, widely entertained among women, that defor-

mities were inherited" is denounced in the *Times*, April 5, 1916, 5, under the headline "Falling Birth-Rate."

107. "Roehampton: The House of Redemption," *Graphic*, November 1916. Margaret Chute (b. 1886) went on to become a columnist for *Picture Show* in the late 1920s.

108. As reported in the *Manchester Evening Chronicle*, clipping dated May–June 1918. The *London Evening Standard* appeal raised over £11,000.

109. Quoted in Pound, *Gillies*, 39.

110. Little, *Artificial Limbs*, 22.

111. Pound, *Gillies*, 27, 29. Gillies and Millard, *Principles and Art of Plastic Surgery*, 10 (where a "Hindu cast of potters" is credited with the discovery of plastic surgery). Albee also compared his work to that of the sculptor, *A Surgeon's Fight*, 109.

112. "Mending the Broken Soldier," *Times* (London), August 12, 1916, 9.

Chapter 3

1. A second official home front photographer, G. P. Lewis, was appointed by the Ministry of Information in April 1918. The main biographical sources on Nicholls are Buckland, *Golden Summer*; Carmichael, "Home Front 1914–18" and *First World War Photographers*; Powell, "Levels of Truth"; and Stearn, "Nicholls."

2. The catalog sequence runs from Q.30.448 to Q.30.459.

3. The Machine Gun Corps Memorial was unveiled in 1925. Aside from Muir's book, a contemporary account of Wood's work at the Third London General Hospital is given in McKenzie, *Reclaiming the Maimed*, 117–24. The other main source is Wood's 1917 article for *The Lancet*. See also Macdonald (*Roses of No Man's Land*, 150–54), which draws on interviews with nurses, doctors, orderlies, and veterans, and Crellin, "Hollow Men."

4. Macdonald, *Roses of No Man's Land*, 150–54. See also Muir, *Happy Hospital*, 23. Wood did in fact make at least one mask for a female civilian who had been treated for an extensive facial ulcer. Her case is documented in Wood, "Masks," 951.

5. The Queen's Hospital, Sidcup, had its own masks unit. See Crellin, "Hollow Men," 80, for a brief discussion of John Edwards's work there.

6. Wood, "Masks," 949.

7. Wood, "Masks," 951. McKenzie similarly emphasizes the role of "sculptural skill" and "imagination" (*Reclaiming the Maimed*, 124).

8. Wood, "Masks," 951.

9. Cruise et al., "Plates for Masking Facial Wounds," 328.

10. Guyatt, "Better Legs," 312–15.

11. In the opening sentence of his *Lancet* article, Wood makes it clear that "no attempt is made in any of my contrivances for the alleviation of the sufferings of the wounded, [or] to restore functioning." The only practical benefit was that wadding placed inside a mask could be used to absorb the discharge from defective tear ducts or salivary glands ("Masks," 949).

12. Wood, "Masks," 949.

13. *The Times History of the War*, vol. 7: 345. The source of *The Times* article is Cruise et al., "Plates for Masking Facial Wounds."

14. *The Times History of the War*, vol. 8: 358.

15. Photographs of the prosthesis, spectacles, and dental plate are available on the online catalog of the museum and archive collections at the Royal College of Surgeons of England: http://surgicat.rcseng.ac.uk, accessed June 19, 2016.

16. Veale's case is illustrated in the article ("Facial Restoration," *Ash's "Quarterly Circular"*).

17. Barry Reay (*Watching Hannah*) borrows the term "monstrous feminine" from Creed, *The Monstrous-Feminine*.

18. *The Diaries and Letters of Arthur J. Munby and Hannah Cullwick*, vol. 1: 12–14. Quoted in Reay, *Watching Hannah*, 39.

19. The first French edition of *Les Œuvres d'Ambroise Paré* appeared in 1575. The "Traitant des moyens et artifices d'adiouster ce qui defaut naturellement ou par accident" is the seventeenth of twenty-nine books.

20. Paré, quoted in Gibson, "Prostheses of Ambroise Paré," 3; and Gilman, *Making the Body Beautiful*, 63.

21. Paré, quoted in Gibson, "Prostheses of Ambroise Paré," 5.

22. Leroux, *The Phantom of the Opera* (2013), 31, 175.

23. Muir, *The Happy Hospital*, 147–48.

24. Muir, *The Happy Hospital*, 152.

25. The British Association of Plastic, Reconstructive and Aesthetic Surgeons (BAPRAS) has a nasal prosthesis made by Henry Brooks for himself, and two ocular prostheses, probably also made by Brooks between 1920 and 1940. An optical technician, Brooks ran a facial prosthetic service at Queen Mary's Hospital Roehampton for thirty years. A mask made at Sidcup by the dental technician Archie Lane was displayed in the *War and Medicine* exhibition: this and two others (one unfinished) are owned by Lane's grandson.

26. Anna Ladd describes the masks as temporary in several of the press clippings in the Archives of American Art. See, for example, "Built New Faces on Wounded Men," March 5, 1919, and "Makes Maimed Faces New," March 6, 1919. Anna Coleman Ladd Papers, box 2, scrapbook, 1914–1923 (folder 5 of 7). Given that the men often underwent multiple operations over several years, this is plausible. Ladd does not, however, explain how some of the masks came into her possession after the war.

27. Nicholson reassured his superiors that "all photographs taken by Mr Nicholls will be submitted for censorship." Memo from Nicholson to Willson, August 2, 1917. MoI Papers, box 3, War Office, IWM file no. 17: Horace W. Nicholls, Ref. 9.

28. Sanders and Taylor, *British Propaganda*, 155.

29. Buckland, *Golden Summer*, 122–23, 128.

30. Buckland, *Golden Summer*, 127–28.

31. Buckland, *Golden Summer*, 127.

32. The figure mentioned in DoI correspondence is £350 per year, although it is possible Nicholls received somewhat less than that following an objection from Willson. Correspondence between Ivor Nicholson, Willson and Masterman, June 26 and 27, 1917. MoI Papers, box 3, War Office, IWM file no. 17: Horace W. Nicholls, Ref. 5 & 6.

33. MoI Papers, box 3, War Office, IWM file no. 17: Horace W. Nicholls, Ref. 3.

34. Buckland, *Golden Summer*, 139.

35. Edwards, "Photography, Materiality and the Performance of the Past."

36. Gower, Jast and Topley, *Camera as Historian*.

37. Edwards, "Straightforward and Ordered."

38. Edwards, "Photography, Materiality and the Performance of the Past."

39. Edwards, "Straightforward and Ordered," 186.

40. Ladd knew about Wood's work from several sources: *The Lancet* article was available in America, and she had a copy of Ward Muir's piece on the Masks for Facial

Disfigurements Department, published in the October 1917 issue of *The Nineteenth Century*. It is also possible that she visited both the Third London General and the Queen's Hospital during the year she spent in Paris. Among her papers is a small notebook containing the address of Captain F. Derwent Wood and directions to the Queen's Hospital for Facial Injuries at Frognal.

41. Ladd kept the letter from Hind, dated September 24, 1917. AAA, ACL Papers, box 2, scrapbook, 1914–1923, folder 5 of 7.

42. The photographs are in the Anna Coleman Ladd Papers, box 2, Scrapbook, 1914–1923. Additional photographs of the Paris studio can be found under "France—Mutilés" in the Library of Congress Prints and Photographs Online Catalogue.

43. Penelope Curtis, foreword to Feeke and Curtis, *Second Skin*.

44. Edouard Papet, "Historical Life Casting," in Feeke and Curtis, *Second Skin*, n.p.

45. Poupelet's contribution is often overlooked in contemporary reports of Anna Coleman Ladd's work in Paris. For an account of their collaboration, see Mitchell, "Facing Horror."

46. The sculpture, and a photograph of Poupelet in the Paris studio, is reproduced in Alain Verstichel, *Sur la Sellette*, March 22, 2011, http://alainverstichel.canal-blog.com/archives/2011/03/22/20698427.html, accessed June 19, 2016.

47. Mitchell, "Facing Horror," 40.

48. According to Ladd, the studio produced five masks for American soldiers and spent about a month on each mask.

49. Mitchell, "Facing Horror," 40–41.

50. Romm and Zacher, "Anna Coleman Ladd," 108.

51. *Sunday Post*, February 16, 1919. Clipping in the Anna Coleman Ladd Papers, AAA, box 2, Scrapbook, 1914–1923 (folder 4 of 7).

52. Mitchell, "Facing Horror," 44.

53. The film, which seems to have been made for distribution in France, is mentioned in official American Red Cross correspondence cited in Romm and Zacher, "Anna Coleman Ladd," 108.

54. Ladd, quoted in Padraic King, "How Wounded Soldiers Have Faced the World Again with Portrait Masks," *St. Louis Post-Dispatch Sunday Magazine*, March 26, 1933. Clipping in the Anna Coleman Ladd Papers, AAA, box 2, Scrapbook, 1914–1923 (folder 4 of 7).

55. "Artist Made Masks for Soldiers," *Philadelphia Press*, March 5, 1919. Clipping in the Anna Coleman Ladd Papers, AAA, box 2, Scrapbook, 1914–1923 (folder 4 of 7).

56. Muriel Caswall, "Woman Who Remade Soldiers' Injured Faces Reaches Boston Home," February 16, 1919. Clipping in the Anna Coleman Ladd Papers, AAA, box 2, Scrapbook, 1914–1923 (folder 4 of 7).

57. David M. Lubin, "Masks, Mutilation and Modernity," 14.

58. Lubin, "Masks, Mutilation and Modernity," 12. Claudine Mitchell argues similarly that the masks "effectively worked to conceal the magnitude of horror." Mitchell, "Facing Horror," 45.

59. Goffman, *Stigma*, 66.

60. Goffman, *Stigma*, 66.

61. *The Concise Oxford Dictionary* (1990) has thirteen entries under "mask."

62. Goffman, *Stigma*, 126.

63. Goffman, *Stigma*, 126.

64. The expression "dreadful abyss" is from the *London Evening Standard*, "Men Shattered in the War," June 1918.

65. Gillies and Millard, *Principles and Art of Plastic Surgery*, 27.

66. Ladd, quoted in Padraic King, "How Wounded Soldiers Have Faced the World Again with Portrait Masks."

67. Pliny the Elder, *Natural History*, 336–37.

68. Charles H. Hart's *Browere's Life Masks of Great Americans* credits Verocchio with the invention of life casting.

69. Cennino d'Andrea Cennini, *The Craftsman's Handbook*, 126.

70. Liz Bruchet, "Unlikely Objects in the Archive," *Slade Archive Project* blog, March 6, 2013, http://blogs.ucl.ac.uk/slade-archive-project/2013/03/06/unlikely-objects-in-the-archive/, accessed June 19, 2016.

71. Hart, *Browere's Life Masks*, quoted in David Meschutt et al., "Life Masks and Death Masks," 315. Hart is less enthusiastic about death masks, remarking, "I have yet to see a death mask that I could recognize by sight."

72. See Feeke and Curtis, *Second Skin*, n.p.

73. Krauss, "Notes on the Index," in *The Originality of the Avant-Garde*, 211.

74. Quoted in Musée d'Orsay, "Second Skin: Life Casting in the 19th Century" (October 2001—January 2002), http://www.musee-orsay.fr/en/events/exhibitions/in-the-musee-dorsay/exhibitions-in-the-musee-dorsay-more/article/a-fleur-de-peau-le-moulage-sur-nature-au-xixe-siecle-4183.html?S=&tx_ttnews[backPid]=649&cHash=daacbd3655&print=1&no_cache=1&, accessed June 19, 2016.

75. "If the artist only reproduces superficial features like a photographer, if he exactly records the diverse features of a physiognomy, but without relating these to character, he does not deserve our admiration. The resemblance he should achieve is that of the soul. Only this matters. This is what the sculptor or painter must seek behind the mask." Rodin, *Art*, 54.

76. Romm and Zacher, "Anna Coleman Ladd," 105.

77. Ladd, quoted in Padraic King, "How Wounded Soldiers Have Faced the World Again with Portrait Masks."

78. Liddle Collection, GS 0790, Holtzapffel, J.G. Typescript recollections and related papers.

79. Lady Kennett, *Self-Portrait of an Artist*, 144.

80. Lady Kennett, *Self-Portrait of an Artist*, October 5, 1918, 167.

81. Lady Kennett, *Self-Portrait of an Artist*, November 4, 1918, 168.

82. Papet, "Historical Life Casting," in Feeke and Curtis, *Second Skin*, n.p. The Slade was the first art school to offer life drawing to female students.

83. Feeke, "Contemporary Sculpture," in Feeke and Curtis, *Second Skin*, n.p.

84. Feeke, "Contemporary Sculpture," in Feeke and Curtis, *Second Skin*, n.p.

85. Erving Goffman, "Embodied Information in Face-to-Face Interaction," *Behavior in Public Places: Notes on the Social Organization of Gatherings*, in Fraser and Greco, *The Body: A Reader*, 85.

86. I owe this analogy to Margaret Collins, consultant orthodontist at Barts and the London Hospitals. The use of silversmiths is mentioned in Mitchell, "Facing Horror," 41.

87. One might therefore question Feo's emphasis on the "discomfort" and "ultimate impracticality" of the masks." See Feo, "Invisibility," 23–24.

88. "I hold over their heads the great power I possess," wrote Wood of his patients: "In three strokes of my wizard's brush I can present to the public such a vision." From a letter to Hamo Thornycroft, dated January 29, 1916 (Henry Moore Institute Archives, C 757), quoted in Koureas, *Memory, Masculinity and National Identity*, 140.

Long associated with illusionistic art, "wizardry" also appears in the cultural lexicon of plastic surgery, as in this passage from the autobiography of American surgeon Max Thorek: "If soldiers whose faces had been torn away by bursting shell on the battlefield could come back into an almost normal life with new faces created by the wizardry of the new science of plastic surgery, why couldn't women whose faces had been ravaged by nothing more explosive than the hand of the years find again the firm contours of youth?" Thorek, *A Surgeon's World*, 164, quoted in Haiken, "Plastic Surgery," 430.

89. Mitchell, "Facing Horror," 45.

Chapter 4

1. A selection of the portraits appeared in the exhibition *Henry Tonks: Art and Surgery* curated by Emma Chambers (Strang Print Room, UCL, October 2002–March 2003).

2. Thanks to Andrew Bamji's archival research, it has been possible to name most of the men whose portraits are reproduced here. I am also very grateful for access to the extensive digital archive that Bamji compiled.

3. Hone notes that Tonks would spend from one to four hours at an operation, mainly taking notes; the diagram would be produced later (*Henry Tonks*, 129).

4. Henry Tonks, Imperial War Museum file, item 18, August 18, 1917.

5. In the past decade the Tonks portraits have featured in *Future Face* at the Science Museum (October 2004–February 2005); *War and Medicine* at Wellcome Collection (November 2008–February 2009); and *Faces of Battle* at the National Army Museum in London (November 2007–August 2008). In June 2007 the full series was made digitally available on the website of the Gillies Archives: http://www.gilliesarchives.org.uk/Tonks%20pastels/index.html, accessed June 19, 2016.

6. Kennett, *Self-Portrait of an Artist*, 144.

7. Tonks, "Notes from 'Wander-Years,'" 223.

8. Quoted in Hone, *Henry Tonks*, 114–15.

9. Quoted in Hone, *Henry Tonks*, 126–26.

10. The comment is attributed to an unnamed "London hostess" by Pound, *Gillies*, 30.

11. Pound, *Gillies*, 30.

12. Quoted in Hone, *Henry Tonks*, 127.

13. Pound, *Gillies*, 26.

14. The photographs were reproduced in a German textbook lent to Gillies by the American dental surgeon Bob Roberts. Pound, *Gillies*, 28.

15. Gillies, quoted in Pound, *Gillies*, 28.

16. Pound, *Gillies*, 28. The American surgeon Fred Albee also compared his work to that of the sculptor (*A Surgeon's Fight*, 109): "Facial reconstruction amounts essentially to sculpturing with live tissues for material. . . . [O]ne must combine mechanical dexterity with artistic feeling."

17. Gillies, quoted in Pound, *Gillies*, 27.

18. Gillies quoted in Bamji, "Facial Surgery," 495.

19. "Face Restoring—Wonders of War Surgery," *Morning Post*, January 1920. London Metropolitan Archives, HO2/QM/Y01/05.

20. In her 2009 article on the Tonks pastels, Emma Chambers pursues questions of subjectivity and spectatorship via psychoanalytic theory. This chapter, in

contrast, emphasizes the cultural and professional contexts of Tonks's collaboration with Gillies.

21. Tonks, "Wander-Years," 223.

22. The expression "necessary Inhumanity" comes from Hunter's introductory lecture to students, ca. 1780, St Thomas's Hospital Manuscript 55, Royal College of Surgeons, 182 verso. Quoted in Richardson, *Death, Dissection and the Destitute*, 31.

23. Bosanquet, "Health Systems in Khaki," 456.

24. Lindsay, "Sir Richard Stawell Oration," 62.

25. Amirault, "Early Medical Photography," 55.

26. O'Connor, "Camera Medica," 232.

27. O'Connor, "Camera Medica," 232.

28. O'Connor, "Camera Medica," 234.

29. There was no formal assessment of the psychological impact of facial injury or reconstructive surgery. The anecdotal evidence for depression is discussed in chapter 2.

30. Carol Armstrong's review of Georges Didi-Huberman's *Invention of Hysteria: Charcot and the Photographic Iconography of the Salpêtrière* provides a critical introduction to this topic: "Probing Pictures: Carol Armstrong on Georges Didi-Huberman," *Artforum International* (September 1, 2003), online version: http://www.thefreelibrary.com, accessed June 19, 2016.

31. O'Connor, "Camera Medica," 234.

32. In addition to works already cited (Amirault, Armstrong, Didi-Huberman, O'Connor), the following titles address aspects of nineteenth-century medical photography: Hamilton and Hargreaves, *The Beautiful and the Damned*; Kemp, "A Perfect and Faithful Record"; McGrath, *Seeing Her Sex*; and the special issue of *History of Photography* on photography, science, and medicine, 23.3 (Autumn 1999).

33. Ludmilla Jordanova's work on the visual cultures of medicine provides the best point of departure in this endeavor. See, for example, "Medicine and Visual Culture"; "Happy Marriages and Dangerous Liaisons"; and *Defining Features*, 11–47.

34. O'Connor refers to the work of John Tagg, Sander Gilman, and Stanley Joel Reiser, among others. "Camera Medica," 233. Patrizia di Bello's study of Victorian women's albums is a notable exception to this historiographical tendency, in its attention to the tactile, imaginative, and social pleasures afforded by collecting and displaying photographs.

35. Cartwright, *Screening the Body*, xv.

36. "Truth in History. Creighton Lecture by Lord Haldane," *Times* (London), March 6, 1914, 9. The quotes that follow are from this article.

37. On photography in World War I, see Carmichael, *First World War Photographers*, and Taylor, *War Photography*.

38. Malvern, *Modern Art, Britain and the Great War*, 49.

39. Jan Gordon, "Art and the Camera," *New Witness*, December 21, 1916, quoted in Malvern, *Modern Art*, 48.

40. Chambers, "Fragmented Identities"; Hone, *Henry Tonks*; Lubbock, "Doing Damage"; Bennett, "Henry Tonks and Plastic Surgery"; and Freeman, "Professor Tonks: War Artist."

41. Hone, *Henry Tonks*, 127.

42. Bennett, "Henry Tonks and Plastic Surgery."

43. Bennett, "Henry Tonks and Plastic Surgery," 14.

44. Gillies, *Plastic Surgery of the Face*, x.

45. Hone, *Henry Tonks*, 128.

46. Bennett, "Henry Tonks and Plastic Surgery," 15.

47. Freeman, "Professor Tonks: War Artist," 289.

48. Freeman, "Professor Tonks: War Artist," 286.

49. Lubbock, "Doing Damage," 58–61.

50. Lubbock, "Doing Damage," 60.

51. Chambers, *Henry Tonks*, 15–16. She expands on this comment in "Fragmented Identities," 589–98.

52. Tonks, quoted in Hone, *Henry Tonks*, 128.

53. Tonks, "Wander-Years," 230.

54. Tonks, "Wander-Years," 224.

55. Charles Blanc, *Grammaire des arts du dessin* (1867), quoted in Callen, *Spectacular Body*, 125.

56. Callen, *Spectacular Body*, 125.

57. Callen, *Spectacular Body*, 125.

58. Chambers mentions that Tonks had favored pastel for life drawing and portraiture since around 1913. "Fragmented Identities," 586.

59. The face-to-face encounter between artist and sitter also distinguishes Tonks's portraits from the photographs and Lindsay's illustrations. Chambers notes the "consensual interaction of looks" implicit in the portraits ("Fragmented Identities," 597), but it is unlikely that Tonks's sitters were in a position to say no. Military rank, class, and personality (formidable in Tonks's case) must have shaped these encounters.

60. Chambers, *Henry Tonks*, 12–13, 41.

61. Extract from an article by Sir Claude Phillips on the New English Art Club, dated December 3, 1915. Tonks correspondence file, Imperial War Museum, London, file no. 300/7, item 96.

62. Callen, *Spectacular Body*, 136.

63. Woodall, *Portraiture*, 8.

64. Tonks quoted in Hone, *Henry Tonks*, 127.

65. Van Alphen, "The Portrait's Dispersal," 239.

66. Tonks, quoted in Chambers, *Henry Tonks*, 13.

67. Morris, *Henry Tonks and the Art of Pure Drawing*, 14.

68. Monnington in Morris, *Henry Tonks*, 15.

69. Chambers argues similarly that the sight of the underface in Tonks's portraits "interrupts the conventional relationship between external and internal identity in portraiture by interposing a fleshy interior between face and self." "Fragmented Identities," 593. Chambers develops this insight with reference to Julia Kristeva's writing on abjection, and Didier Anzieu's concept of the "skin ego."

70. Correspondence quoted in Morris, *Henry Tonks*, 37.

71. Tonks, quoted in Bennett, "Henry Tonks and Plastic Surgery," 15; and in "Dickie Orpen on Henry Tonks," *Dickie Orpen: Surgeons' Artist*, 5. Diana Orpen (1914–2008) was the daughter of William Orpen. Both were taught by Tonks at the Slade, Dickie when she was only fifteen. During World War II she followed Tonks's example, producing drawings of reconstructive surgery at the Plastic and Maxillo-Facial Unit at Hill End St Albans. Her drawings are in the collection of the British Association of Plastic, Reconstructive and Aesthetic Surgeons (BAPRAS).

72. "Art boy" was Tonks's dismissive term for critics. See Chaplin, *Slade School of Fine Art Archive Reader*, part 7.6 (unpaginated). See also Cast, "Representing Reality.

73. Cast, "Representing Reality," 293–94.

74. Cast, "Representing Reality," 291–92.

75. Chambers, "Cultivation of Mind and Hand," 99.

76. Cast, "Representing Reality," 291; Chambers, "Cultivation of Mind and Hand," 102.

77. Fothergill was Tonks's student from 1905 to 1909. I have used his essay as my main source for Tonks's ideas about drawing, as Tonks himself wrote very little on the subject (the few exceptions, mostly from letters, are glossed in Hone and Morris), nor did he produce any statements for the school's calendar or annual reports (Chaplin, *Slade School of Fine Art Archive reader*, vol. 2, n.p.). Given the official nature of Fothergill's publication, Chambers thinks it likely that "the ideas expressed in this article are very close to those of Tonks himself" (*Henry Tonks*, 25 n. 14). A similar assessment is made by Chaplin, who identifies Fothergill's sources as Tonks's "informal instruction in the life room" and conversations with other students (6.44).

78. Fothergill, "Teaching Drawing at the Slade," 34.

79. Fothergill, "Teaching Drawing at the Slade," 47.

80. Fothergill, "Teaching Drawing at the Slade," 38 n. 1.

81. Fothergill, "Teaching Drawing at the Slade," 42.

82. Gillies, *Plastic Surgery of the Face*, 4–6.

83. Gillies, *Plastic Surgery of the Face*, 49.

84. Fothergill, "Teaching Drawing at the Slade," 41.

85. "The word 'snapshot' is a hateful word and is only fit for a photographer," Tonks wrote in a letter to the Girls' Public Day School Trust in November 1909 (quoted in Morris, *Henry Tonks*, 29).

86. Chaplin, *Slade School of Fine Art Archive reader*, 7.7.

87. Chaplin, *Slade School of Fine Art Archive reader*, 7.7.

88. Tonks, quoted in Morris, *Henry Tonks*, 21.

89. Hone, *Henry Tonks*, 43.

90. The exhibition catalog *Henry Tonks and the Art of Pure Drawing*, edited by Lynda Morris, includes the reminiscences of some of Tonks's students, including David Bomberg, Thomas Monnington, Helen Lessore, and William Coldstream. Tonks also taught Lewis, Nash, Nevinson, and Stanley Spencer, among others, in the first two decades of the century: relationships that were often intensely competitive. He makes a brief and unlikable appearance in Nash's autobiography: *Outline*, 89–91, 93. For a fictionalized account of the war experiences of this generation of Slade students, see Pat Barker's *Life Class* and *Toby's Room*.

91. C. R. W. Nevinson, "How the War Vindicated Modern Methods in Art," Tate Gallery Archive, 7311.2, item 34, cited in Corbett, *Modernity of English Art*, 48.

92. Corbett, *Modernity of English Art*, 14.

93. Corbett, *Modernity of English Art*, 8.

94. Tickner, *Modern Life and Modern Subjects*, 189.

95. Tonks, quoted in Cast, "Representing Reality," 294.

96. Lessore in Morris, *Henry Tonks*, 8.

97. Callen, *Spectacular Body*, 136.

98. Gustave Geffroy, *La Justice*, May 26, 1886, quoted in Callen, *Spectacular Body*, 136.

Chapter 5

1. Jordanova, "Happy Marriages and Dangerous Liaisons," 101.

2. For a recent reassessment, see Lanchester, "Is It Art?"

3. Jordanova, "Happy Marriages and Dangerous Liaisons," 101.

4. Jordanova, "Happy Marriages and Dangerous Liaisons," 112.

5. Launched in April 2007 by Joanna Ebenstein, a Brooklyn-based graphic designer and photographer, the *Morbid Anatomy* website is devoted to "the interstices of art and medicine, death and culture."

6. Game Rankings: http://www.gamerankings.com/, accessed February 8, 2011. The *BioShock II* website claims more than fifty game-of-the-year awards for the franchise. http://2kgamesinternational.com/uk/games/bioshock2/.

7. http://www.2kgames.com/#/news/2k-games-announces-first-installment-of-bioshock-reg-2-downloadable-content-now-available, accessed February 8, 2011.

8. http://www.gilliesarchives.org.uk/Tonks%20pastels/index.html, accessed February 8, 2011.

9. Pat Barker and Suzannah Biernoff, "Art in Conflict" podcast, LSE, March 2, 2013, http://www.lse.ac.uk/publicEvents/events/2013/03/LitFest20130302t-1300vSZT.aspx.

10. Project Façade: www.projectfacade.com, accessed February 8, 2011; *Faces of Battle*, November 2007–August 2008, National Army Museum, London; *War and Medicine*, November 2009—February 2009, Wellcome Collection, London.

11. Visitors' book entry for November 13, 2007.

12. Visitors' book entry for June 15, 2008.

13. Visitors' book entry for November 11, 2007.

14. Allbutt was regius professor at Cambridge from 1892 until his death in 1925. This quote is from Brain, "Facial Surgery during World War I," 157.

15. Cooter, "War and Modern Medicine," 1544.

16. Cooter, "War and Modern Medicine," 1553.

17. Albee, *A Surgeon's Fight*, 93–94, 106.

18. During World War I, 82 percent of "wounded" British troops and 93 percent of the "sick" were eventually returned to duty. Cooter, "War and Modern Medicine," 1541.

19. http://www.projectfacade.com/index.php?/case/C81/, http://www.project-facade.com/index.php?/galleries/comments/lumley, http://www.gilliesarchives.org.uk/Tonks%20pastels/content/tonks67_lumley_large.html, accessed October 1, 2009.

20. The relevant records are WO 372: Medal Index Card entry; WO 339/57830: Officers' service records; and MH 106/2204: Medical Sheets: Royal Flying Corps, I–O. I am grateful to Paddy Hartley of Project Façade for this information.

21. Canadian Libraries Internet Archive: http://www.archive.org/details/plastic-surgeryof00gilluoft, accessed February 8, 2011.

22. Sontag, *On Photography*, 20.

23. Sontag, *Regarding the Pain of Others*, 6.

24. Sontag, *Regarding the Pain of Others*, 16.

25. Sontag, *Regarding the Pain of Others*, 79.

26. Sontag, *Regarding the Pain of Others*, 80.

27. Sontag, *Regarding the Pain of Others*, 91.

28. Sontag, *Regarding the Pain of Others*, 102. The phrase "let the atrocious images haunt us" appears in Sontag's prefatory essay for a 2001 book of Don McCullin's photographs. Under the title "Witnessing" the essay concludes: "A photograph can't coerce. It won't do the moral work for us. But it can start us on the way."

29. Sontag acknowledges the influence of Brink and Zelizer. *Regarding the Pain of Others*, 107.

30. Sontag, *Regarding the Pain of Others*, 107.

31. Sontag, *Regarding the Pain of Others*, 74.

32. The "Face of War" photographs in Friedrich's book are mentioned several times: see 13–14 and 37.

33. Sontag, *Regarding the Pain of Others*, 37–38.

34. In a 2009 study of responses to the portrayal of disfigurement on television, focus group participants spoke of disfigurement as a "last taboo" compared to the representation of other minority groups (Wardle and Boyce, "Media Coverage and Audience Reception," 4).

35. Face Equality information leaflet (London: Changing Faces, 2008).

36. Wardle and Boyce, *Media Coverage and Audience Reception*, 137.

37. Tagg, *Burden of Representation*, 64.

38. 2K Forums, "Project Façade vs BioShock?" July 18–23, 2007: http://forums.2kgames.com/forums/archive/index.php/t-1836.html, accessed June 19, 2016.

39. The link to the concept art is now inactive, but the artwork is reproduced in the *BioShock* players' manual (Walsh, *BioShock*, 51). Examples can also be seen on the *BioShock* wiki: http://bioshock.wikia.com/wiki/Toasty, accessed February 8, 2011.

40. In Lumley's case there are no known relatives. In order to protect the privacy of the other families, no identifying details have been included here.

41. 2K Forums, "Project Façade vs BioShock?" July 18, 2007, 11:51 p.m.

42. 2K Forums, "Project Façade vs BioShock?" July 18, 2007, 12:37 a.m., 12:45 a.m.

43. 2K Forums, "Project Façade vs BioShock?" July 19, 2007, 10:28 a.m.

44. 2K Forums, "Project Façade vs BioShock?" July 19, 2007, 01:17 p.m.

45. 2K Forums, "Project Façade vs BioShock?" July 19, 2007, 01:28 p.m.

46. 2K Forums, "Project Façade vs BioShock?" July 19, 2007, 02:29 p.m.

47. 2K Forums, "Project Façade vs BioShock?" July 20, 2007, 01:02 p.m.

48. The term "ethics" is used here (as in the OED) to refer to a set of moral principles or rules concerning human conduct. Both ethics and morality are taken to be sociohistorical formations. In this, my approach differs from much of the philosophical literature on ethics.

49. Sicart, *Ethics of Computer Games*, 17.

50. Sicart, *Ethics of Computer Games*, 3.

51. Sicart, *Ethics of Computer Games*, 228. Pornography is mentioned here too, as deserving of further study, particularly in light of cultural preferences and prohibitions. Sicart notes that "Japanese pornographic games could scandalize any given European culture, while Western role-playing games are often deemed uninteresting in Japan."

52. The literary references most often mentioned by reviewers are George Orwell and Ayn Rand, the latter embodied in the game by Rapture's megalomaniac creator, the business magnate Andrew Ryan.

53. Joe McDonagh interviewed by Patrick Kolan, IGN AU. "AU BioShock Q&A: The Moral Dilemma," http://uk.pc.ign.com/articles/798/798746p1.html, accessed February 8, 2011.

54. Copyright law places the onus on the user to make a reasonable effort to locate the copyright holder. In the case of Project Façade, each page of the website carried the copyright line © Paddy Hartley. Hartley subsequently added the disclaimer (which also appears on the Gillies Archives website): "The medical images which

appear on this site . . . are not to be reproduced or used for professional or commercial purposes without the express permission of the [Gillies] archive."

55. *Bioshock Making Of* (view from 5:50): http://www.youtube.com/watch?v=FQ7YT8Ajr0c, accessed February 8, 2011. Wells credits Ken Levine with the discovery of Project Façade.

56. For an interesting parallel, see Jones, "Makeover Culture's Dark Side."

57. BioShock Medical Pavilion trailer, YouTube, http://www.youtube.com/watch?v=Qw_9sAqmDtI, accessed October 10, 2013.

58. Gunning, "Cinema of Attractions." Although the term was coined as a description of early cinema (1895–1906), Adam Lowenstein argues for its usefulness in analyzing the "attractions" of horror films in "Living Dead."

59. Weise, "Bioshock," 153.

60. BioShock wiki, "Limits of Imagination," http://bioshock.wikia.com/wiki/Limits_of_Imagination, accessed October 10, 2013.

61. BioShock wiki, "Surgery's Picasso," http://bioshock.wikia.com/wiki/Surgery%27s_Picasso, accessed October 10, 2013.

62. BioShock wiki, "Toasty," http://bioshock.wikia.com/wiki/Toasty, accessed October 10, 2013.

63. Deitch *Post Human*, np.

64. Boss, "Vile Bodies," 20.

65. Boss, "Vile Bodies," 19.

66. On Leonardo da Vinci's *Grotesque Heads*, see Clark, *Leonardo*, 120–24; Gombrich, "Grotesque Heads" in *The Heritage of Apelles*; and Clayton, *Leonardo*.

67. Bell, "Francis Bacon," 2007.

68. The conversation took place on December 7, 2009, at the Wellcome Trust, London.

69. Wellcome Library, Archives and Manuscripts RAMC 760. The photographs were taken by Dr. Albert Norman, Honorary Scientific Photographer, between 1916 and 1918.

70. The public part of the database is divided into "historical" and "contemporary" images. A third category—clinical images—is password protected and restricted to registered users (mostly doctors, public health officials, and medical publishers). Wellcome Images also does specific searches on behalf of commercial clients. Where a patient can be identified, his or her permission is required before a photograph can be published.

71. Catherine Draycott, email correspondence, December 17, 2009.

72. "Project Façade vs BioShock?" not_john_galt, July 19, 2007, 1. 23 pm. That *BioShock* deals in "moral grey areas" is a claim made repeatedly in reviews and publicity. In a preview on Yahoo Games, for example, Ken Levine promises "plenty of moral ambiguity. . . . We wanted a different system than the typical dark side/light side thing. . . . For us, it's all grey side." July 3, 2007, http://videogames.yahoo.com/printview_feature?eid=523932, accessed December 1, 2009.

73. 2K Forums, "Project Façade vs BioShock?" July 19, 2007, 12:44 am.

74. 2K Forums, "Project Façade vs BioShock?" July 19, 2007, 01:03 am.

75. The lecture can be downloaded from the GDC website. The distressed breathing is at 32:20–33:35.

76. Kahn, *Heraclitus*, 256–59.

77. Sekula, "Reading an Archive," 445.

78. Sekula "The Body and the Archive," 7.

79. Cross and Peck, editorial, 128.

80. Cross and Peck, editorial, 128.

81. Jameson, *Postmodernism*, 27–28.

82. *BioshockMakingOf*(viewfrom5:50):http://www.youtube.com/watch?v=FQ7YT8Ajr0c, accessed February 8, 2011.

83. Coleman, "Ethnographic Approaches," 488.

84. Price, *Dispersion*, n.p. Both an essay and an artwork, *Dispersion* exists, appropriately enough, in multiple versions: as a downloadable pdf; a series of wall-mounted panels; and a printed booklet.

85. For Price, "the readymade still towers over artistic practice."

86. Wesch, "YouTube," 21.

87. Wesch, "YouTube," 23.

88. Wesch, "YouTube," 28–29.

89. Sontag, *Regarding the Pain of Others*, 37, 108.

90. Sontag, *Regarding the Pain of Others*, 109.

91. Sontag, *Regarding the Pain of Others*, 108.

92. Interestingly, the Science Museum in London does take account of "cultural objections or taboos surrounding the representation of remains, as well as the display of remains themselves." However, this sensitivity extends only to images of non-European remains. http://www.sciencemuseum.org.uk/about_us/about_the_museum/collections/human_remains/human_remains_policy.aspx, accessed February 8, 2011.

Conclusion

1. Aside from Barker's novel, the Queen's Hospital features in Conny Braam's *The Cocaine Salesman* and Louisa Young's *My Dear, I Wanted to Tell You*.

2. Bamji, "Facial Surgery," 500.

3. Bamji, "Facial Surgery," 500.

4. *What Are You Staring At?* BBC2, August 6, 2003. Hutchison's comment was quoted on the BBC website *Ouch!* a few days later, August 11, 2003: http://www.bbc.co.uk/ouch/features/what_are_you_staring_at_968.shtml,accessed June 19, 2016. He also appeared on BBCi for a live chat following the broadcast of the documentary. An edited transcript is available on *Ouch!*, http://www.bbc.co.uk/ouch/features/ouch_home_837.shtml, August 11, 2003.

5. Scarry, *On Beauty*, 74, 16, quoted in Schweik, *Ugly Laws*, 286.

6. James Partridge, "Image Conscience," interview in the *Guardian*, May 2, 2007: http://www.theguardian.com/society/2007/may/02/health.guardiansocietysupplement, accessed June 19, 2016.

7. By this I mean ways of seeing as well as social attitudes and stereotypes. Standard definitions of the social model usually stress environmental and organizational (as well as attitudinal) barriers to inclusion. See, for example, the UK Office for Disability Issues website: http://odi.dwp.gov.uk/about-the-odi/the-social-model.php, accessed December 17, 2013.

8. "By definition," Goffman writes, "we believe the person with a stigma is not quite human" (*Stigma*, 15, 24).

9. "Interaction-uneasiness" (Goffman's term) is discussed in chapter 1.

10. Sontag, *Regarding the Pain of Others*, 68.

11. Siebers, *Disability Aesthetics*, 2–3.

12. Siebers, *Disability Aesthetics*, 4.

13. Siebers cites André Breton's ideal of "convulsive beauty" in his introduction (4) and discusses the Russian formalist technique of *ostranenie* ("defamiliarization") in relation to medical photography (44–6). Hal Foster's "The Return of the Real" is mentioned in a chapter on trauma art (112–13). The concepts of abjection and "wound culture" are equally relevant to many of Siebers's examples from the 1990s onward. See, in particular, Kristeva, *Powers of Horror* and Seltzer, *Serial Killers*; and for a critique of the aesthetics of abjection, Jay, "Abjection Overruled."

14. Butler, *Precarious Life*, 146 (quoted in full in chapter 1).

15. Turner, "Social Fluids," 1, 6. Turner is discussed at greater length in the introduction.

16. Lady Kennet, *Self-Portrait of an Artist*, 168.

17. Siebers, *Disability Aesthetics*, 103.

18. Mitchell in Smith, *Visual Culture Studies*, 36.

Works Cited

Archives

Anna Coleman Ladd Papers, Archives of American Art (AAA).
Art Department and Photograph Archive, Imperial War Museum, London (IWM).
The Gillies Archives, Queen Mary's Hospital Sidcup.
Liddle Collection, University of Leeds.
London Metropolitan Archives, Clerkenwell, London (LMA).

Historical Sources

Albee, Fred H. *A Surgeon's Fight to Rebuild Men: An Autobiography*. London: Robert Hale, 1950.

Bacon, Roger. *The Opus Majus of Roger Bacon*. Translated by R. B. Burke. 2 vols. New York: Russell, 1962.

Cennino d'Andrea Cennini. *The Craftsman's Handbook: The Italian "Il Libro Dell'Arte."* Translated by Daniel V. Thompson. New York: Dover, 1960.

Cruise, Richard, Somerville Hastings, and Derwent Wood. "Plates for Masking Facial Wounds." *Journal of Royal Army Medical Corps* 26 (January–June 1916): 324–29.

Darwin, Leonard (Major). "The Disabled Sailor and Soldier and the Future of Our Race." *Eugenics Review* 9 (1917): 1–17.

Dostoyevsky, Fyodor. *The Idiot*. Translated by David Magarshack. New York: Penguin, 1955.

"Facial Restoration." *Ash's "Quarterly Circular"* (September 1896): 1–8.

Fothergill, John. "The Principles of Teaching Drawing at the Slade." In *The Slade*, ed. Fothergill, 31–47. London: Slade School, University College, 1907.

Galsworthy, John. Foreword to *Handbook for the Limbless*, edited by G. Howson, v–vi. London: Disabled Society, 1922.

Galsworthy, John. "The Gist of the Matter." *Reveille* 1 (1918): 3–19.
Gillies, Harold D. *Plastic Surgery of the Face Based on Selected Cases of War Injuries of the Face Including Burns, with Original Illustrations.* London: Frowde, Hodder and Stoughton, 1920.
Gillies, Harold D., and D. Ralph Millard. *The Principles and Art of Plastic Surgery.* London: Butterworth, 1957.
Glubb, John. *Into Battle: A Soldier's Diary of the Great War.* London: Cassell, 1978.
Gower, H. D., J. Stanley, and W. W. Topley. *The Camera as Historian.* London: Sampson Low, Marston, 1916.
Hart, Charles H. *Browere's Life Masks of Great Americans.* New York: Doubleday, 1899.
Hutchinson, Jonathan. *Syphilis.* London: Cassell, 1887.
Lady Kennet [Kathleen, Lady Scott]. *Self-Portrait of an Artist: From the Diaries and Memoirs of Lady Kennet.* London: John Murray, 1949.
Leroux, Gaston. *The Phantom of the Opera.* Translated by Alexander Teixeira de Mattos. London: Mills & Boon, 1911.
Leroux, Gaston. *The Phantom of the Opera.* London: Fantastica, 2013.
Lindsay, Daryl. "The Sir Richard Stawell Oration." *Medical Journal of Australia,* 45th year, 1.3 (January 18, 1958): 61–65.
Lombroso, Gina. *The Tragedies of Progress.* Translated by C. Taylor. New York: E. P. Dutton, 1931.
McKenzie, Robert Tait. *Reclaiming the Maimed: A Handbook of Physical Therapy.* New York: Macmillan, 1918.
Muir, Ward. *The Happy Hospital.* London: Simpkin, Marshall, 1918.
Muir, Ward. *Observations of an Orderly: Some Glimpses of Life and Work in an English War Hospital.* London: Simpkin, Marshall, 1917.
Nash, Paul. *Outline: An Autobiography and Other Writings.* London: Faber and Faber, 1949.
Pliny the Elder. *Natural History: A Selection.* Translated by John Healey. London: Penguin Classics, 2004.
Rodin, Auguste. *Art: Conversations with Paul Gsell.* Translated by Jacques de Caso and Patricia B. Sanders. Berkeley: University of California Press, 1984.
Service, Robert W. *Rhymes of a Red Cross Man.* Toronto: W. Briggs, 1916.
Thorek, Max. *A Surgeon's World: An Autobiography.* Philadelphia: J. B. Lippincott, 1943.
The Times History of the War. 22 vols. 1914–21.
Tonks, Henry. "Notes from 'Wander-Years.'" *Artwork* 5.20 (1929): 213–35.
Wood, Francis Derwent. "Masks for Facial Wounds." *The Lancet,* June 23, 1917, 949–51.

Secondary Sources

Adams, Parveen. *The Emptiness of the Image: Psychoanalysis and Sexual Differences.* London: Routledge, 1996.
Amirault, Chris. "Posing the Subject of Early Medical Photography." *Discourse* 16.2 (Winter 1993–94): 51–76.
Apel, Dora. "Cultural Battlegrounds: Weimar Photographic Narratives of War." *New German Critique* 76 (1999): 49–84.
Apel, Dora. *War Culture and the Contest of Images.* New Brunswick: Rutgers University Press, 2012. Kindle edition.

Bakhtin, Mikhail. *Rabelais and His World.* Translated by Hélène Iswolsky. Bloomington: Indiana University Press, 1984.

Bamji, Andrew. "The Art of Medicine: Faces of War." *The Lancet*, March 2, 2013, 718–19.

Bamji, Andrew. "Facial Surgery: The Patient's Experience." In *Facing Armageddon: The First World War Experienced*, edited by Hugh Cecil and Peter H. Liddle, 490–501. London: Leo Cooper, 1996.

Barker, Pat. *Life Class.* London: Hamish Hamilton, 2007.

Barker, Pat. *Toby's Room.* London: Hamish Hamilton, 2012.

Barthes, Roland. *A Lover's Discourse: Fragments.* Translated by Richard Howard. London: Vintage, 2002.

Bell, Julian. "The Cunning of Francis Bacon." *New York Review of Books* 54.8 (May 10, 2007). http://www.nybooks.com/articles/20150

Bennett, J. P. "Henry Tonks and Plastic Surgery." *Supplement to the British Journal of Plastic Surgery* 39 (1986): 1–34.

Berman, Nina. *Homeland.* London: Trolley Books, 2008.

Berman, Nina. *Purple Hearts: Back from Iraq.* London: Trolley Books, 2004.

Biernoff, Suzannah. *Sight and Embodiment in the Middle Ages.* Basingstoke: Palgrave, 2002.

Bourdieu, Pierre. *Distinction: A Social Critique of the Judgement of Taste.* Translated by Richard Nice. London: Routledge, 1984.

Bogdan, Robert. "The Social Construction of Freaks." In *Freakery: Cultural Spectacles of the Extraordinary Body*, edited by Rosemarie Garland-Thomson, 23–37. New York: New York University Press, 1996.

Bosanquet, Nick. "Health Systems in Khaki: The British and American Medical Experience." In *Facing Armageddon: The First World War Experienced*, edited by Hugh Cecil and Peter H. Liddle, 451–65. London: Leo Cooper, 1996.

Boss, Pete. "Vile Bodies and Bad Medicine." *Screen* 27 (January 1986): 14–25.

Bourke, Joanna. *Dismembering the Male: Men's Bodies, Britain and the Great War.* London: Reaktion, 1996.

Braam, Conny. *The Cocaine Salesman.* Translated by Jonathan Reeder. London: Haus Publishing, 2011.

Brain, David J. "Facial Surgery during World War I." *Facial Plastic Surgery* 9.2 (April 1993): 157–64.

Brink, Cornelia. "Secular Icons: Looking at Photographs from Nazi Concentration Camps." *History and Memory* 12.1 (2000): 135–50.

Buci-Glucksmann, Christine. *Baroque Reason: The Aesthetics of Modernity.* London: Sage, 1994.

Buckland, Gail. *The Golden Summer: The Edwardian Photographs of Horace W. Nicholls.* London: Pavilion, 1989.

Butler, Judith. *Frames of War: When Is Life Grievable?* New York: Verso, 2009.

Butler, Judith. *Precarious Life: The Powers of Mourning and Violence.* London: Verso, 2004.

Callen, Anthea. *The Spectacular Body: Science, Method and Meaning in the Work of Degas.* New Haven: Yale University Press, 1995.

Callister, Sandy. "'Broken Gargoyles': The Photographic Representation of Severely Wounded New Zealand Soldiers." *Social History of Medicine* 20 (2007): 111–30.

Carden-Coyne, Ana. *Reconstructing the Body: Classicism, Modernism and the First World War.* Oxford: Oxford University Press, 2009.

Carmichael, Jane. *First World War Photographers*. London: Routledge, 1989.
Carmichael, Jane. "Home Front 1914–18: The Photographs of G. P. Lewis and Horace Nicholls." *Creative Camera* 247–48 (1985): 58–63.
Cartwright, Lisa. *Screening the Body: Tracing Medicine's Visual Culture*. Minneapolis: University of Minnesota Press, 1995.
Cast, David. "Representing Reality: G. E. Moore, Tonks, Coldstream, Victor Pasmore and Others." *Word and Image* 16.3 (1985): 290–95.
Chambers, Emma. "The Cultivation of Mind and Hand: Teaching Art at the Slade School of Fine Art 1868–92." In *Governing Cultures: Art Institutions in Victorian London*, edited by Paul Barlow and Colin Trodd, 98–113. Aldershot: Ashgate, 2000.
Chambers, Emma. "Fragmented Identities: Reading Subjectivity in Henry Tonks' Surgical Portraits." *Art History* 32.3 (2009): 578–607.
Chambers, Emma. *Henry Tonks: Art and Surgery*. London: College Art Collections, University College London, 2002.
Chaplin, Stephen. *A Slade School of Fine Art Archive Reader: A Compendium of Documents, 1868–1975, in University College London, Contextualised with an Historical and Critical Commentary, Augmented with Material from Diaries and Interviews*. London: UCL, 1998.
Clark, Kenneth. *Leonardo da Vinci*. Harmondsworth: Penguin, 1989.
Clayton, Martin. *Leonardo da Vinci: The Divine and the Grotesque*. London: Royal Collection Enterprises, 2002.
Cohen, Deborah. *The War Came Home: Disabled Veterans in Britain and Germany, 1914–39*. Berkeley: University of California Press, 2001.
Cole, Jonathan. *About Face*. Cambridge, MA: MIT Press, 1999.
Coleman, E. Gabriella. "Ethnographic Approaches to Digital Media." *Annual Review of Anthropology* 39 (2010): 487–505.
Connor, J. T. H., and Michael Rhode. "Shooting Soldiers: Civil War Medical Images, Memory and Identity in America." *Invisible Culture* 5 (2003): 1–15.
Cooter, Roger. *Surgery and Society in Peace and War: Orthopaedics and the Organization of Modern Medicine*. London: Macmillan, 1993.
Cooter, Roger. "War and Modern Medicine." In *Companion Encyclopaedia of the History of Medicine*, edited by W. F. Bynum and Roy Porter, vol. 1, 1536–73. London: Routledge, 1993.
Corbett, David Peters. *The Modernity of English Art, 1914–30*. Manchester: Manchester University Press, 1997.
Creed, Barbara. *The Monstrous-Feminine: Film, Feminism, Psychoanalysis*. London: Routledge, 1993.
Crellin, Sarah. "Hollow Men: Francis Derwent Wood's Masks and Memorials, 1915–25." *Sculpture Journal* 6 (2001): 75–87.
Cross, Karen, and Julia Peck. "Editorial: Special Issue on Photography, Archive and Memory." *Photographies* 3.2 (2010): 127–38.
Das, Santanu. *Touch and Intimacy in First World War Literature*. Cambridge: Cambridge University Press, 2005.
Davis, Keith F. "'A Terrible Distinctiveness': Photography of the Civil War Era." In *Photography in Nineteenth-Century America*, edited by Martha A. Sandweiss, 131–79. New York: Harry N. Abrams, 1991.
Davis, Lennard J. "Introduction: Normality, Power, and Culture." In *The Disability Studies Reader*, 4th ed., edited by Lennard J. Davis. New York: Routledge, 2013.

Deitch, Jeffrey, ed. *Post Human*. Cantz/Deste Foundation for Contemporary Art, 1992.

Di Bello, Patrizia. *Women's Albums and Photography in Victorian England: Ladies, Mothers and Flirts*. Aldershot: Ashgate, 2007.

Dickie Orpen: Surgeons' Artist. London: Camberwell College of Arts / Royal College of Surgeons, 2008–9.

Eco, Umberto, ed. *On Ugliness*. London: Harvill Secker, 2007.

Edwards, Elizabeth. "Straightforward and Ordered: Amateur Photographic Surveys and Scientific Aspiration, 1885–1914." *Photography and Culture* 1.2 (2008): 185–210.

Edwards, Elizabeth. "Unblushing Realism and the Threat of the Pictorial: Photographic Survey and the Production of Evidence, 1885–1918." *History of Photography* 33.1 (2009): 3–17.

Feeke, Stephen, and Penelope Curtis. *Second Skin: Historical Life Casting and Contemporary Sculpture*. Leeds: Henry Moore Institute, 2002.

Foster, Hal. *The Return of the Real*. Cambridge, MA: October Books / MIT Press, 1996.

Foucault, Michel. *The Birth of the Clinic: An Archaeology of Medical Perception*. Translated by A. M. Sheridan Smith. London: Routledge, 2003.

Foucault, Michel. *Discipline and Punish: The Birth of the Prison*. Translated by Alan Sheridan. London: Allen Lane, Penguin, 1977.

Fox, Paul. "Confronting Post-war Shame in Weimar Germany: Trauma, Heroism and the War Art of Otto Dix." *Oxford Art Journal* 29 (2006): 247–67.

Fraser, Mariam, and Monica Greco, eds. *The Body: A Reader*. Abingdon: Routledge, 2005.

Freeman, Julian. "Professor Tonks: War Artist." *Burlington Magazine*, May 1985, 285–93.

Gerber, David A., ed. *Disabled Veterans in History*. Ann Arbor: University of Michigan Press, 2000.

Gibson, Thomas. "The Prostheses of Ambroise Paré." *British Journal of Plastic Surgery* 8 (1955–56): 3–8.

Gilman, Sander. *Making the Body Beautiful: A Cultural History of Aesthetic Surgery*. Princeton: Princeton University Press, 1999.

Gogh, Paul. *A Terrible Beauty: War, Art and the Imagination, 1914–18*. Bristol: Sansom, 2009.

Goffman, Erving. *Stigma: Notes on the Management of Spoiled Identity*. London: Penguin, 1968.

Gombrich, E. H. *The Heritage of Apelles: Studies in the Art of the Renaissance*. Oxford: Phaidon, 1976.

Gunning, Tom. "The Cinema of Attractions: Early Film, Its Spectator and the Avant-Garde." In *Early Cinema: Space Frame Narrative*, edited by Thomas Elsaesser, 56–62. London: BFI, 1990.

Guyatt, Mary. "Better Legs: Artificial Limbs for British Veterans of the First World War." *Journal of Design History* 14 (2001): 307–25.

Haiken, Beth. "Plastic Surgery and American Beauty at 1921." *Bulletin of the History of Medicine* 68 (1994): 429–53.

Hamilton, Peter, and Roger Hargreaves. *The Beautiful and the Damned: The Creation of Identity in Nineteenth Century Photography*. London: Lund Humphries and National Portrait Gallery, 2001.

Hirschhorn, Michelle. "Orlan: Artist in the Post-human Age of Mechanical Reincarnation: Body as Ready (to Be Re-) Made." In *Generations and Geographies in the Visual Arts: Feminist Readings*, edited by Griselda Pollock, 110–34. London: Routledge, 1996.

Hone, Joseph. *The Life of Henry Tonks.* London: Heinemann, 1939.

Iversen, A. C., et al. "Risk Factors for Post-traumatic Stress Disorder among UK Armed Forces Personnel." *Psychological Medicine* 38 (2008): 511–22.

James, Sarah. "Making an Ugly World Beautiful? Morality and Aesthetics in the Aftermath." In *Memory of Fire: Images of War and the War of Images*, edited by Julian Stallabrass, 114–29. Brighton: Photoworks, 2013.

Jameson, Frederic. *Postmodernism, or, The Cultural Logic of Late Capitalism.* Durham, NC: Duke University Press, 1990.

Jay, Martin. "Abjection Overruled." In Jay, *Cultural Semantics*, 144–56. London: Athlone Press, 1998.

Johansen, Jorgen Dines. *Signs in Use: An Introduction to Semiotics.* New York: Routledge, 2002.

Jones, Meredith. "Makeover Culture's Dark Side: Breasts, Death and Lolo Ferrari." *Body and Society*, special issue "Surgery and Embodiment." 14.1 (2008): 89–104.

Jordanova, Ludmilla. *Defining Features: Scientific and Medical Portraits, 1660–2000.* London: Reaktion / National Portrait Gallery, 2000.

Jordanova, Ludmilla. "Happy Marriages and Dangerous Liaisons: Artists and Anatomy." In *The Quick and the Dead: Artists and Anatomy*, 100–113. London: Hayward Gallery, 1997.

Jordanova, Ludmilla. "Medicine and Visual Culture." *Social History of Medicine* 3.1 (1990): 89–99.

Kahn, Charles H. *The Art and Thought of Heraclitus: An Edition of the Fragments with Translation and Commentary.* Cambridge: Cambridge University Press, 1979.

Katovsky, Bill, and Timothy Carlson. *Embedded: The Media War in Iraq.* Guilford, CT: Lyons Press, 2003.

Kemp, Martin. "A Perfect and Faithful Record: Mind and Body in Medical Photography before 1900." In *Beauty of Another Order*, edited by Ann Thomas, 120–49. New Haven: Yale University Press, 1997.

Koureas, Gabriel. *Memory, Masculinity and National Identity in British Visual Culture, 1914–1930.* Aldershot: Ashgate, 2007.

Koven, Seth. "Remembering and Dismemberment: Crippled Children, Wounded Soldiers, and the Great War in Great Britain." *American Historical Review* 99.4 (1994): 1167–202.

Krauss, Rosalind E. *The Originality of the Avant-Garde and Other Modernist Myths.* Cambridge, MA: MIT Press, 1986.

Kristeva, Julia. *Black Sun: Depression and Melancholia.* Translated by Leon S. Roudiez. New York: Columbia University Press, 1989.

Lanchester, John. "Is It Art?" *London Review of Books*, January 1, 2009, 18–20.

Linker, Beth. *War's Waste: Rehabilitation in World War I America.* Chicago: University of Chicago Press, 2011.

Lowenstein, Adam. "Living Dead: Fearful Attractions of Film." *Representations* 110 (Spring 2010): 105–28.

Lubbock, Tom. "Doing Damage." *Modern Painters* 12.1 (1999): 58–61.

Lubin, David M. "Masks, Mutilation and Modernity: Anna Coleman Ladd and the First World War." *Archives of American Art Journal* 47 (Fall 2008): 4–15.

Macdonald, Lyn. *The Roses of No Man's Land.* London: Michael Joseph, 1980.

McCullin, Don. *Don McCullin*. London: Jonathan Cape, 2001.

McGrath, Roberta. *Seeing Her Sex: Medical Archives and the Female Body*. Manchester: Manchester University Press, 2002.

Malvern, Sue. *Modern Art, Britain and the Great War*. New Haven: Yale University Press, 2004.

Mandler, Peter. "The Problem with Cultural History." *Cultural and Social History* 1.1 (2004): 94–117.

Merleau-Ponty, Maurice. *The Primacy of Perception*. Evanston, IL: Northwestern University Press, 1964.

Meschutt, David, et al. "Life Masks and Death Masks." *American Journal of Forensic Medicine and Pathology* 13.4 (1992): 315–19.

Meyer, Jessica. *Men of War: Masculinity and the First World War*. London: Palgrave, 2009.

Mitchell, Claudine. "Facing Horror: Women's Work, Sculptural Practice, and the Great War." In *Work and the Image*, vol. 2, *Work in Modern Times: Visual Meditations and Social Processes*, edited by Valerie Mainz and Griselda Pollock, 33–53. London: Ashgate, 2000.

Morris, Lynda, ed. *Henry Tonks and the Art of Pure Drawing*. Norwich: Norwich School of Art Gallery, 1985.

Nessen, Shawn Christian, Dave Edmond Lounsbury, and Stephen P. Hetz. *War Surgery in Afghanistan and Iraq: A Series of Cases, 2003–2007*. Falls Church, VA: Office of the Surgeon General / Borden Institute, 2008.

Newman, Kathy. "Wounds and Wounding in the American Civil War: A Visual History." *Yale Journal of Criticism* 6.2 (1993): 63–86.

Nicolson, Juliet. *The Great Silence: 1918–1920, Living in the Shadow of the Great War*. London: John Murray, 2009.

O'Connor, Erin. "Camera Medica: Towards a Morbid History of Photography." *History of Photography* 23.3 (1999): 232–44.

Park, Katharine, and Lorraine J. Daston. "Unnatural Conceptions: The Study of Monsters in Sixteenth- and Seventeenth-Century France and England." *Past and Present* 92 (August 1981): 20–54.

Peirce, Charles S. "Logic as Semiotic: The Theory of Signs." In *The Philosophical Writings of Peirce*, edited by Justus Buchler. New York: Dover, 1955.

Perry, Heather R. "Re-arming the Disabled Veteran: Artificially Rebuilding State and Society in World War One Germany." In *Artificial Parts, Practical Lives: Modern Histories of Prosthetics*, edited by Katherine Ott, David Serlin, and Stephen Mihm, 75–101. New York: New York University Press, 2002.

Pound, Reginald. *Gillies, Surgeon Extraordinary*. London: Michael Joseph, 1964.

Powell, R. "Levels of Truth: The Life and Work of Horace Nicholls." *British Journal of Photography* 128.27 (1981): 672–74.

Price, Seth. *Dispersion*. 2002–. http://www.distributedhistory.com/Disperzone.html. Accessed February 8, 2011.

Reay, Barry. *Watching Hannah: Sexuality, Horror and Bodily De-formation in Victorian England*. London: Reaktion, 2002.

Reznick, Jeffrey. *Healing the Nation: Soldiers and the Culture of Caregiving in Britain during the Great War*. Manchester: Manchester University Press, 2005.

Reznick, Jeffrey. "Prostheses and Propaganda: Materiality and the Human Body in the Great War." In *Matters of Conflict: Material Culture, Memory and the First World War*, edited by Nicholas J. Saunders, 51–61. London: Routledge, 2004.

Richardson, Ruth. *Death, Dissection and the Destitute*. London: Routledge, 1987.

Romm, Sharon, and Judith Zacher. "Anna Coleman Ladd: Maker of Masks for the Facially Mutilated." *Plastic and Reconstructive Surgery* 70.1 (1982): 104–11.
Russo, Mary. *The Female Grotesque: Risk, Excess and Modernity.* London: Routledge, 1997.
Sanders, Michael L., and Philip M. Taylor. *British Propaganda during the First World War, 1914–18.* London: Macmillan, 1982.
Schweik, Susan M. *The Ugly Laws: Disability in Public.* New York: New York University Press, 2009.
Seib, Philip. *Beyond the Front Lines: How the News Media Cover a World Shaped by War.* New York: Palgrave Macmillan, 2004.
Sekula, Allan. "The Body and the Archive." *October* 39 (1986): 3–64.
Sekula, Allan. "Reading an Archive: Photography between Labour and Capital." In *The Photography Reader,* edited by Liz Wells, 443–52. London: Routledge, 2003.
Seltzer, Mark. *Serial Killers: Death and Life in America's Wound Culture.* London: Routledge, 1998.
Sennett, Richard. *The Fall of Public Man.* New York: Norton, 1974.
Shaw, Philip. "'Disgusting Objects:' Images of Wounding in the Aftermath of War." In *Suffering and Sentiment in Romantic Military Art,* 175–210. London: Ashgate, 2013.
Shilling, Chris. *The Body and Social Theory.* London: Sage, 1993.
Sicart, Miguel. *The Ethics of Computer Games.* Cambridge, MA: MIT Press, 2009.
Siebers, Tobin. *Disability Aesthetics.* Ann Arbor: University of Michigan Press, 2010.
Smith, Marquard. *Visual Culture Studies: Interviews with Key Thinkers.* London: Sage, 2008.
Sontag, Susan. *Illness as Metaphor* and *AIDS and Its Metaphors.* London: Penguin, 1991.
Sontag, Susan. *On Photography.* New York: Penguin, 1977.
Sontag, Susan. *Regarding the Pain of Others.* London: Penguin, 2003.
Stallabrass, Julian, ed. *Memory of Fire: Images of War and the War of Images.* Brighton: Photoworks, 2013.
Stallybrass, Peter, and Allon White. *The Politics and Poetics of Transgression.* London: Methuen, 1986.
Stearn, R. T. "Nicholls, Horace Walter (1867–1941)." *Dictionary of National Biography.* Oxford: Oxford University Press, 2006. http://www.oxforddnb.com/index/101058922/Horace-Nicholls
Tagg, John. *The Burden of Representation: Essays on Photographies and Histories.* Houndmills: Macmillan, 1988.
Taylor, John. *War Photography: Realism in the British Press.* London: Routledge, 1991.
Thomson, Rosemarie Garland, ed. *Freakery: Cultural Spectacles of the Extraordinary Body.* New York: New York University Press, 1996.
Thomson, Rosemarie Garland. *Staring: How We Look.* Oxford: Oxford University Press, 2009.
Tickner, Lisa. *Modern Life and Modern Subjects.* New Haven: Yale University Press, 2000.
Turner, Bryan S. *The Body and Society: Explorations in Social Theory.* Oxford: Blackwell, 1984.
Turner, Bryan S. "Social Fluids: Metaphors and Meanings of Society." *Body and Society* 9.1 (2003): 1–10.
Turner, Bryan S. *Vulnerability and Human Rights.* University Park: Pennsylvania State University Press, 2006.
Turner, Fred. Review of *Alive Day Memories: Home from Iraq. Journal of American History,* June 2008, 288–90.

Twine, Richard. "Physiognomy, Phrenology and the Temporality of the Body." *Body and Society* 8.1 (2002): 67–88.

Van Alphen, Ernst. "The Portrait's Dispersal: Concepts of Representation and Subjectivity in Contemporary Portraiture." In *Portraiture: Facing the Subject*, edited by Joanna Woodall, 239–56. Manchester: Manchester University Press, 1997.

Vetrocq, Marcia. "Rules of Engagement." *Art in America*, June–July 2008, 168–75, 208–9.

Walsh, Doug. *BioShock*. Bradygames Signature Series Guide. Indianapolis: DK Publishing, 2007.

Wardle, Claire, and Tammy Boyce. *Media Coverage and Audience Reception of Disfigurement on Television*. 2009. www.cardiff.ac.uk/jomec/resources/09mediacoverageofdisfigurement.pdf

Wehbi, Samantha. "Representing Disability and Disfigurement: Modes of Representation in Nina Berman's Photographs." *Disability Studies Quarterly* 32.1 (2012): http://dsq-sds.org/article/view/3035

Weise, Matthew Jason. "Bioshock: A Critical Historical Perspective." *Eludamos* 2.1 (2008): 151–55.

Wesch, Michael. "YouTube and You: Experiences of Self-Awareness in the Context Collapse of the Recording Webcam." *Explorations in Media Ecology* 8.2 (2009): 19–34.

Winter, Jay. *Sites of Memory, Sites of Mourning: The Great War in European Cultural History*. Cambridge: Cambridge University Pres, 1993.

Wombell, Paul. "Face to Face with Themselves: Photography in the First World War." In *Photography/Politics Two*, edited by Patricia Holland, Jo Spence, and Simon Watney, 71–81. London: Routledge, 1987.

Woodall, Joanna, ed. *Portraiture: Facing the Subject*. Manchester: Manchester University Press, 1997.

Woolf, Virginia. *Three Guineas*. Edited by Naomi Black. Oxford: Blackwell, 2001.

Young, Louisa. *My Dear, I Wanted to Tell You*. London: HarperCollins, 2011.

Zelizer, Barbie. *Remembering to Forget: Holocaust Memory through the Camera's Eye*. Chicago: University of Chicago Press, 1998.

Index

abjection, 6, 24, 64, 161, 168, 189n69, 195n13
aesthetics, 5, 9, 24, 62, 64, 65, 118, 127, 153, 167–69, 195n13. *See also* beauty; ugliness
aesthetic surgery, 14, 65, 71, 107–8. *See also* plastic surgery
Afghanistan, war, 25, 27–29, 37, 49, 141
Albee, Fred, 56, 141, 178n4, 187n16
Alive Day Memories: Home From Iraq (HBO), 28–30, 32–33, 40, 51, 141, 167–68
American Civil War: medical photographs, 18, 173n72
American Red Cross, 20, 99–102
Amirault, Chris, 123
amputees, 24, 28, 30, 32–34, 57, 60, 74, 76–78, 182n106. *See also* disability; prosthetic limbs
antibiotics, 179n17
Apel, Dora: *War Culture and the Contest of Images*, 31–32, 34, 37, 51
archives. *See* Gillies Archives; photographic archives
Archives of American Art, 99–104, 184n26
art education, 110, 117, 132–37, 186n82. *See also* Slade School of Fine Art; Tonks
Atlas-Manuel des maladies de la bouche, 154–55
aversion, 8, 10, 20, 63, 56, 59, 96, 147, 169. *See also* disgust; horror; stigma

Bacon, Francis, 13, 56, 127, 154–55, 162; *Three Studies for Figures at the Base of a Crucifixion*, 154
Bacon, Roger, 15
Bakhtin, Mikhail: *Rabelais*, 16–17. *See also* grotesque
Bamji, Andrew, 60, 66, 69, 140, 164–65. *See also* Gillies Archives
Barker, Pat: *Life Class*, 190n90; *Toby's Room*, 140, 164, 190n90, 194n1
Barthes, Roland: reality effect, 14, 126, 158
Battle of the Somme, 13, 118
Battle of Waterloo, 18, 27
beauty, 15, 17, 42, 63–65, 69, 105, 113, 116, 129, 162, 165–66, 172n43; alternative ideas of, 24, 136–37, 168–69, 195n13; critique of beauty, 53; cult of beauty, 8. *See also* aesthetics; aesthetic surgery; classical tradition
Beckmann, Max, 19. *See also* Weimar Germany
Bell, Charles: Battle of Waterloo watercolours, 18, 27

Berman, Nina, 1–3, 8, 14, 17–18, 32, 34–35, 40–43, 46, 50–54, 58, 167–68; *Marine Wedding*, 1–3, 5, 17, 40–43, 50–53; *Purple Hearts: Back from Iraq*, 17, 34–36, 40, 46, 50–51, 53
Biernoff, Suzannah: *Sight and Embodiment in the Middle Ages*, 4
BioShock, 5, 8, 22, 139, 148–53, 155–59, 161–63, 168; concept art, 148–50, 159, 192n39; copyright, 150, 156–57, 192n54; discussion forum, 5, 148, 156, 161; *Making of BioShock*, 152; medical themes, 152–53, 157; score, 22, 157–58
Blackwell, Geoffrey, 117
Blanc, Charles: *Grammaire des arts du dessin*, 129
blindness and visual impairment, 28, 41–42, 71, 75, 87–91, 97, 103, 105–6, 180n52
Body Shock, 16
Bogdan, Robert, 16
Boss, Pete, 154
Bourdieu, Pierre: physical capital, 40, 71
Bourke, Joanna: *Dismembering the Male*, 5–6, 8–9, 62, 71, 76, 166
breath, 22, 157–58, 161, 163
Brighton Photo Biennial, 38–39
British Association of Plastic, Reconstructive and Aesthetic Surgeons (BAPRAS), 184n25, 189n71
British Red Cross, 67, 117, 130
Brooke Army Medical Center, Texas, 1, 34
Brooks, Henry, 184n25
Buckland, Gail, 97
Butler, Judith, 31–32, 37–38, 54; *Bodies That Matter*, 11; *Frames of War*, 31–32; *Precarious Life*, 25, 37–38

Callen, Anthea: *Spectacular Body*, 129, 131
Callister, Sandy, 178n7
Cambridge Military Hospital, Aldershot, 68, 71–72, 117–19, 128
Carden-Coyne, Ana: *Reconstructing the Body*, 5–8, 10
carnivalesque, 16
Cartwright, Lisa: *Screening the Body*, 125
Cennini, Cennino: *Il Libro Dell'Arte*, 108
censorship, 7–8, 20, 28, 57, 96, 105, 169; self-censorship, 7, 57
Chambers, Emma, 128–29, 187n20, 189n69, 190n77; *Henry Tonks: Art and Surgery*, 21, 167, 187n1
Changing Faces, 147, 166
Christian iconography, 4, 38, 60–65, 129–31, 179n22. *See also* icon; sacrifice
classical tradition, 4–6, 17, 30, 65, 67, 110, 131, 169, 173n67
Cole, Jonathan: *About Face*, 57
Compton, Martyn, 48–49, 168
computer games: ethics of, 22, 148–52, 155–57; realism in, 138, 156–59. *See also BioShock*
context: collapse, 159–63; contexts of viewing, 22, 24, 31, 41, 116, 125, 146; definitions of, 139, 159–60
Cooter, Roger, 141
Corbett, David Peter: *Modernity of English Art*, 135–36
corporeal history, 5, 8; *The Body: A Reader*, 10–11, 13–14, 16
cosmetic surgery. *See* aesthetic surgery
Cross, Karen, 158
Cullwick, Hannah, 89
cultural imaginary, 7

The Dark Knight (film), 13
Das, Santanu, 7
Daston, Lorraine, 15
death, representations of, 4, 7, 17, 30, 60–62, 64, 108, 172n44
Deeks, Charles, 120–24
Degas, Edgar, 129, 131, 133, 136
depression, 21, 74–76, 180n47, 182n91, 188n29
digital media, 22, 27, 157, 159–60. *See also* computer games; context collapse
disability, 7, 19, 23–24, 32, 41–42, 50, 78, 147, 166, 171n11, 174n97, 177n68, 181n69; disability aesthetics, 167–69, 179n18; medical and social models, 9, 166, 168, 194n7. *See also* amputees; stigma
Disability Discrimination Act (UK), 166

disfigurement: as an "aesthetic error," 65; artistic representations of, 19, 24, 64, 167–69 (*see also* Bell; Tonks); disfiguring effects of syphilis, 59, 64–65, 88–89, 165, 179n17; female cases, 71, 89–90, 101–2, 183n4; horror of, 4, 9, 16, 18, 60, 73, 165; idealized feminine gaze and touch, 58–59; as "last taboo," 9; as loss of humanity, 13, 15, 19, 40, 57–58, 106, 119; loss of identity, 15, 57, 71, 80, 169; medical and social models, 9, 165–66; pensions, 66, 71, 181n69; pity, 16, 58, 72, 76; psychological impact, 66, 74–76, 188n29; as "worst loss of all," 19, 69. *See also* aversion; facial injury; masks; plastic surgery; stigma
disgust, 64, 71, 136. *See also* aversion
Dix, Otto, 19, 127. *See also* Weimar Germany
drawing: compared to photography, 114, 116, 119, 123–25, 127–29, 134–35, 140, 162, 167–68; and tactility, 132–37. *See also* pastel; Tonks

Eco, Umberto: *On Ugliness*, 64–65
Edwards, Elizabeth, 98
Edwards, John, 183n5
embarrassment, 56
emotions. *See* aversion; disgust; embarrassment; empathy; horror; pity; shame
empathy, 3, 24, 48, 50–51, 59, 142, 169
ethics: definition, 192n48; and computer games, 148–52, 155–56, 161, 163, 193n72; of spectatorship, 24, 144, 146–47, 165, 169, 191n28
Evans, Reginald, 67–69
exhibitions, 1, 21, 116, 126–27, 140, 146, 161, 182n89; *Faces of Battle*, 21, 140–41, 174n83, 187n5; *Future Face*, 21, 187n5; *Henry Tonks and the Art of Pure Drawing*, 190n90; *Henry Tonks: Art and Surgery*, 21, 167, 187n1; *The Quick and the Dead: Artists and Anatomy*, 138–39; *Second Skin: Historical Life Casting and Contemporary Sculpture*, 110, 112; *War and Medicine*, 21, 53, 140, 184n25, 187n5. *See also* Brighton Photo Biennial; Imperial War Museum

facial injury: first-hand accounts, 66–69, 180n45, 180n53; psychological impact, 66, 74–76, 188n29; in World War I, 7, 15, 18–20, 28, 56, 58–60, 64, 69, 71, 96, 110, 142, 146, 165. *See also* Deeks; Gillies; *Gueules cassées*; Lumley; Nicholls; plastic surgery; Tonks; Wood
Fothergill, John: "Principles of Teaching Drawing," 133–36; 190n77
Foucault, Michel: *Birth of the Clinic*, 47; *Discipline and Punish*, 11–12; influence, 11, 125, 158
Fraser, Mariam: *The Body: A Reader*, 10–11, 13–14, 16
"freaks," 16, 50, 151.
Friedrich, Ernst: *Krieg dem Kriege!*, 146

Galsworthy, John, 76–77, 182n104
Gandolfini, James: *Alive Day Memories*, 28–30
Garland-Thomson, Rosemarie: *Freakery*, 16, 22; *Staring: How We Look*, 23–24
Gillies Archives, 5, 21–22, 60, 119, 124, 140, 146, 148, 159, 165, 192n54
Gillies, Harold Delf, 71, 73, 75, 78, 80, 106, 109, 114, 117–18, 123–24, 127–28, 134, 142, 148, 156, 164, 182n91; *Plastic Surgery of the Face*, 116, 144. *See also* Gillies Archives
Gilman, Sander: *Making the Body Beautiful*, 14–15, 57, 65
Glubb, John, 180n53
Goffman, Erving: *Behavior in Public Places*, 112; *Stigma*, 41–42, 105, 113, 164, 166
The Great Sacrifice, 60–62, 179n22
Greco, Monica: *The Body: A Reader*, 10–11, 13–14, 16
Greenfield-Sanders, Timothy: *Alive Day Memories* portraits, 32–34, 40, 50–51, 167
Griffiths, Stuart, 5, 8, 17–18, 34–37, 40, 42–50, 53–54, 167–68; *Closer*, 44–47, 54, 177n80; *Isolation* (film), 18, 37, 43, 50

grotesque, 11, 15–17, 19, 55, 58, 64, 69, 73, 96, 154, 168
Gueules cassées, 20, 99–105, 113
Guyatt, Mary, 76–77

Halfaker, Dawn, 30, 32–34
Hartley, Paddy: *Faces of Battle*, 21, 140–41, 174n83, 187n5. *See also* Project Façade
Hayward Gallery, London: *The Quick and the Dead: Artists and Anatomy*, 138–39
Headley Court, Surrey, 43
Henry Moore Institute, Leeds: *Second Skin: Historical Life Casting and Contemporary Sculpture*, 110, 112
"heroic individualism," 28, 32, 34, 37
Hind, Lewis, 99, 185n41
history of the body. *See* corporeal history
Holbein, Hans: *Dead Christ*, 63
Holtzapffel, J.G.H., 66–67, 69, 109
Hone, Joseph: *Henry Tonks*, 127, 135, 187n3, 190n77
horror, 3–4, 6, 9, 16, 18, 26, 59, 60, 62–65, 71–73, 80, 113, 146–47, 162, 164–65; films, 153–54
hospitals: in *BioShock*, 152–54, 157; Cambridge Military Hospital, Aldershot, 68, 71–72, 117–19, 128; Hospital du Val-de-Grâce, Paris, 18, 102; John Ellerman Hospital, Regent's Park, 20, 67, 109–10; King George Military Hospital, London, 156; The London Hospital, 116, 128; Queen Mary Auxiliary Hospital, Roehampton, 76–79, 182n96; The Queen's Hospital, Sidcup (later Queen Mary's Hospital), 69–70, 72–73, 75, 114–15, 181n82, 183n5, 194n1; Third London General Hospital, Wandsworth, 19, 56, 58, 71, 75, 81–82, 93, 180n53; Zafaraniah Hospital, Baghdad, 38–39
humanity: concept of, 21, 31, 40, 167; disfigurement as loss of, 13, 15, 19, 40, 57–58, 106, 119; portrayal of, 37–40
Human Tissue Act, 162
Hunter, William, 123
Hutchison, Iain, 165

icon, 39, 146, 162
identity: disfigurement as loss of, 15, 57, 71, 80, 169; and portraiture, 12–13, 37, 40, 52–54, 128, 131, 167, 189n69. *See also* subjectivity
Imperial War Museum, London, 74, 81, 98
Index: theory of, 41, 54, 109, 132, 162
Iraq War, 1, 25–30, 34, 37–39, 48, 51
Isolation (film), 18, 37, 43, 50

Jameson, Frederic: "pastness," 159
James, Sarah, 39–40
John Ellerman Hospital, Regent's Park, 20, 67, 109–10
Jordanova, Ludmilla: *Defining Features*, 40; *The Quick and the Dead: Artists and Anatomy*, 138–39, 161

King George Military Hospital, London, 156
Koureas, Gabriel: *Memory, Masculinity and National Identity*, 7, 9–10, 64
Kristeva, Julia: on Holbein's *Dead Christ*, 63; "symbolic collapse," 21, 60, 179n18

Ladd, Anna Coleman, 20, 99–110, 112–13, 169, 184n26, 184n40
Lane, Archie, 184n25
Leonardo da Vinci: *Grotesque Heads*, 154
leprosy, 15, 64
Leroux, Gaston: *Phantom of the Opera*, 65, 92
Lessore, Helen, 136
Lewis, Percy Wyndham, 126, 135, 190n90
Liddle Collection, 66, 164, 180n45
likeness, 18, 37, 46, 54, 108, 132, 162–63, 178n106. *See also* portraiture
limb loss. *See* amputees
Lindsay, Daryl, 123, 129
Linton, Simi, 42
Lobley, J. Hodgson, 74–75
The London Hospital, 116, 128
Lubbock, Tom, 127–28
Lubin, David, 105

Lumley, Henry, 142–45, 147–50, 156–63, 192n40

MacColl, D. S., 117, 132
Malvern, Sue: *Modern Art, Britain and the Great War*, 126
masks: death masks, 108, 186n71; life masks 107–12; portrait masks, 20, 80–108, 112–13.
McKenzie, Robert Tait, 75, 182n92
medical illustration, 114, 119–20, 123–34, 132, 187n3
medical imaginary, 154
medical photography. *See* photography
Merleau-Ponty, Maurice, 57–58
Merrick, Joseph, 116
"military sublime," 38–39
mirrors, 7, 19, 49, 55, 57, 67
Mitchell, W. J. T., 169
modernism, 127, 135–36, 168
monstrous, 13, 15–16, 64; "monstrous feminine," 89
morality. *See* ethics
Morbid Anatomy, 139, 191n5
Morestin, Hippolyte, 118
Muir, Ward: *Happy Hospital*, 19, 56, 58, 69, 71, 74, 93–96, 166, 184n40
Munby, Arthur J., 89

Nash, Paul, 22, 126, 135, 190n90
National Army Museum, London: *Faces of Battle*, 21, 140–41, 174n83, 187n5
Nevinson, C. R. W., 126–27, 135, 190n90
New Belvedere House, Stepney, 36, 42
New English Art Club, 117
Nicholls, Horace, 20–21, 81–99, 183n1
Nicholson, Ivor, 97–98
Norfolk, Simon, 38–39
nose: artificial, 88–90, 92–95, 105–6, 109; grotesque, 16; missing, 40, 65, 67, 69, 75, 89, 92, 110; rhinoplasty, 14; "Tin Noses Shop," 84
nursing, accounts of, 56, 58–59, 67–68, 72, 179n8

O'Connor, Erin, 124–25
Orlan, 13–14
Orpen, Dickie (Diana), 133, 189n71

Paralympic Games, 24
Paré, Ambroise, 90, 95
Park, Katherine, 15
Partridge, James, 165–66
passing, 15, 105. *See also* stigma
pastel, 20–21, 122, 127–32, 110–11, 114–16, 136, 140
Peck, Julia, 158
pensions. *See* war pensions
Phantom of the Opera, 65, 92
photography: Abu Ghraib photographs, 31; before and after photographs, 13, 95, 121, 134, 173n47; compared to art, 114, 116, 119, 123–25, 126–29, 134–35, 140, 162, 167–68; documentary function, 37, 48, 124–26, 160–61; medical photography, 40, 46, 48, 123–25, 158, 160; photographic archives, 11–12, 56, 81, 98–99, 158–59; photographic survey movement, 98–99; portrait photography, 11–12, 32, 37–40, 47
phrenology, 12
physical capital, 40, 71
physiognomy, 12–13, 65, 89, 94, 172n34, 172n38, 186n75
Picasso, Pablo, 37, 127, 153
pity, 16, 24, 51, 58, 72, 76
plastic surgery: as sculpture, 187n16; in World War I, 118–23, 134, 140–44, 156, 164–65, 187n88. *See also* aesthetic surgery; Gillies; Orlan
portrait masks. *See* masks
portraiture: definitions, 12–13, 40, 50, 53–54, 109, 131–32, 167; and likeness, 18, 37, 46, 54, 108, 132, 162–63, 178n106; portrait masks, 20, 80–108, 112–13; portrait photography, 11–12, 32, 37–40, 47. *See also* Berman; Greenfield-Sanders; Griffiths; Nicholls; Tonks
Pound, Reginald: *Gillies, Surgeon Extraordinary*, 118
Poupelet, Jane, 20, 101–3, 185n45
Poynter, Edward, 133
Price, Seth: *Dispersion*, 159–60
Project Façade, 140–42, 148, 150, 152, 156, 192n54

propaganda, 20, 26, 57, 74, 78, 81, 96, 98, 114, 147
prosthetic limbs, 32–33, 52, 60, 76–80. *See also* amputees
prosthetic masks. *See* masks
PTSD, 43. *See also* facial injury: psychological impact

Queen Mary Auxiliary Hospital, Roehampton, 76–79, 182n96
The Queen's Hospital, Sidcup (later Queen Mary's Hospital), 69–70, 72–73, 75, 114–15, 181n82, 183n5, 194n1

realism, 113, 126–27, 138, 148, 157–58
Reay, Barry: *Watching Hannah*, 89
reconstructive surgery. *See* plastic surgery
Red Cross. *See* American Red Cross; British Red Cross
redemption, 22, 60, 77–78. *See also* Christian iconography
Rodin, Auguste, 101, 109–10, 186n75
Rosenkranz, Karl: *Aesthetics of Ugliness*, 64–65
Royal Army Medical Corps (RAMC), 19, 69, 74–75, 82, 93, 117
Royal College of Surgeons of England, 87, 116, 119, 140, 164

sacrifice, 4, 30, 59–64, 76, 80, 140–41, 165, 179n22, 179n24. *See also* Christian iconography
Scarry, Elaine: *Body in Pain*, 11; *On Beauty*, 165
scars, 41, 45, 49, 59, 69, 74, 118, 127, 133, 144
Schyman, Garry, 157–58, 162
Science Museum, London: *Future Face*, 21, 187n5; human remains policy, 194n92
Scott, Kathleen, 20, 67, 109–10, 116, 169
Sekula, Allan: "The Body and the Archive," 11–12, 47, 158, 172n34
Service, Robert: "Fleurette," 55, 58
shame, 19, 96, 147, 162
Sicart, Miguel: *Ethics of Computer Games*, 151–52, 157, 192n51
Siebers, Tobin: *Disability Aesthetics*, 167–69, 195n13
sight: the gaze, 23, 42, 47, 58–59, 116, 125, 128, 140; spectacle, 16–17, 25, 29, 60, 135, 146, 153; surveillance, 12, 23, 125, 158; visual pleasure, 161. *See also* aversion; staring; visual culture; voyeurism
sin, 15–16, 65
Slade School of Fine Art, London, 20–21, 108–9, 114, 117, 132–33, 186n82, 189n71, 190n77, 190n90
Somme. *See* Battle of the Somme
Sontag, Susan: *Illness as Metaphor*, 64; On *Photography*, 144; *Regarding the Pain of Others*, 3, 31, 144, 146–47, 162, 165, 167
Stallabrass, Julian: *Memory of Fire*, 25–26, 38–39
staring, 23–24, 42, 54, 72, 165
St. Dunstan's Hostel, 180n52
stereotype, 12, 41–42, 58
stigma, 18, 20, 23, 32, 41–42, 48, 58, 65, 92, 105, 113, 147, 165–66, 177n68, 194n8
stoicism, 9, 58, 66, 69, 166
subjectivity, 10, 14, 40, 50, 52, 131–32, 160, 187n20. *See also* identity
surgery: as allegory, 152–54. *See also* aesthetic surgery; plastic surgery; *War Surgery in Afghanistan and Iraq*
syphilis, 59, 64–65, 88–89, 165, 179n17

Tagg, John: *Burden of Representation*, 147, 158
therapeutic idiom, 30, 47
Third London General Hospital, Wandsworth, 19, 56, 58, 71, 75, 81–82, 93, 180n53
Times History of the War, 75, 87, 178n6
Tin Noses Shop, 84
"Toasty" (*BioShock*), 149–50, 153
Tonks, Henry, 20–22, 108–11, 114–23, 126–37, 139–40, 142, 145, 162, 167–69
touch, 7, 58–59, 116, 128, 131, 132–37
Treves, Frederick, 116

tuberculosis, 64, 88
Turner, Bryan: *Body and Society*, 10; "Social Fluids," 4, 19, 168
Turner, Fred, 29–30

ugliness, 11, 24, 42, 54, 64–65, 68, 105, 118, 136, 165–66, 168
University College London (UCL): *Henry Tonks: Art and Surgery*, 21, 167, 187n1. *See also* Slade School of Fine Art

Valadier, Charles Auguste, 118
Val-de-Grâce Hospital, Paris, 18, 102
Vetrocq, Marcia, 32, 50
vision. *See* sight
visual culture, 4–5, 31, 42, 59, 125, 160, 169. *See also* sight
voice, 13–14, 157
voyeurism, 23, 50, 114, 147, 162

Walter Reed Army Medical Center, Washington, D.C., 29, 33–34
War Illustrated, 7, 178n6
war memorials, 5, 21–22, 82, 169, 179n18, 179n22
War on Terror, 28
war pensions, 66, 71, 181n69
War Surgery in Afghanistan and Iraq, 27–29
Wehbi, Samantha, 50
Weimar Germany, 4, 19, 56, 173n76
Wellcome Collection: *War and Medicine*, 21, 53, 140, 184n25, 187n5
Wellcome Images, 156, 193n70
Wellington House, 20, 81, 96, 98, 114
Wesch, Michael, 160
Whitney Biennial, 34, 53
Winter, Jay: *Sites of Memory*, 21–22, 179n18
Wlérick, Robert, 101
Woodall, Joanna: *Portraiture*, 131, 178n106
Wood, Francis Derwent, 20, 80, 82, 84–93, 97, 99, 105–6, 112–13, 167, 183nn3–4,183n11, 186n88
Woolf, Virginia, 3–4
work ethic, 77–78
World Press Photo Contest, 1, 40

YouTube, 152, 160

Ziegel, Tyler, 1, 14, 40–42, 50, 52–53, 58

Printed and bound by CPI Group (UK) Ltd, Croydon, CR0 4YY

16/09/2026

14963491-0003